Reclaiming Your Life After Rape

Cognitive-Behavioral Therapy
For Posttraumatic Stress Disorder

Client Workbook

Barbara Olasov Rothbaum
Edna B. Foa

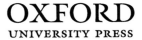

OXFORD
UNIVERSITY PRESS

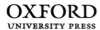

OXFORD
UNIVERSITY PRESS

Oxford University Press, Inc., publishes works that further
Oxford University's objective of excellence
in research, scholarship, and education.

Oxford   New York
Auckland   Cape Town   Dar es Salaam   Hong Kong   Karachi
Kuala Lumpur   Madrid   Melbourne   Mexico City   Nairobi
New Delhi   Shanghai   Taipei   Toronto

With offices in
Argentina   Austria   Brazil   Chile   Czech Republic   France   Greece
Guatemala   Hungary   Italy   Japan   Poland   Portugal   Singapore
South Korea   Switzerland   Thailand   Turkey   Ukraine   Vietnam

ISBN-13 978-0-19-518376-4

Printed in the United States of America
on acid-free paper

Contents

▇ Section III. Cognitive-Behavioral Program
Confronting The Traumatic Memories

Chapter 10: Imaginal Exposure: Reliving the Trauma Memory in Imagination

■ Section IV. Cognitive-Behavioral Program
Stress Management Techniques

■ Section V. Cognitive-Behavioral Program
Putting It All Together

Comments About The Program

Internationally acclaimed authors Rothbaum and Foa present their empirically supported treatment for rape-related PTSD in clear, concise terms. Clients and their clinicians will benefit from the proposed treatment as the methods and the process are clearly explicated. The empirical data firmly support this treatment for women who have been sexually assaulted and develop PTSD. The client workbook represents a breakthrough in the field. It is at once authoritative, precise, and readable. The authors are to be congratulated on another fine contribution to the field of trauma and PTSD.

Terence M. Keane, PhD
Director, National Center for PTSD
VA Boston Healthcare System
Professor and Vice Chairman of Psychiatry
Boston University School of Medicine

Drs. Rothbaum and Foa have developed an extremely helpful Client Workbook. The client workbook provides clients with critical understanding of PTSD and the specific treatment strategies to address avoidance, reexperiencing symptoms, and distortions in thinking related to traumatic events. The workbook is a valuable resource for therapists as well. It includes material geared towards the client that can give the therapist a more in-depth model of how to provide the treatment rationales and to communicate with clients about the treatment strategies and techniques to be used.

The authors bring years of clinical experience and expertise in treatment development and evaluation to the material included in the *Reclaiming Your Life After Rape: Cognitive-Behavioral Therapy For Posttraumatic Stress Disorder* Client Workbook.

Heidi Resnick, PhD
Associate Professor, Clinical Psychology
National Crime Victims Research and Treatment Center
Medical University of South Carolina
Associate Editor, *Journal of Traumatic Stress*

About the Authors

BARBARA OLASOV ROTHBAUM, PHD, received her PhD in clinical psychology from the University of Georgia in 1986 and is currently a tenured associate professor in psychiatry and Director of the Trauma and Anxiety Recovery Program at the Emory University School of Medicine. Dr. Rothbaum specializes in research on the treatment of individuals with anxiety disorders, particularly focusing on exposure therapy, with a specialty in Posttraumatic Stress Disorder (PTSD). She was on the DSM-IV Workgroup on PTSD, has won both state and national awards for her research, has authored over 60 scientific papers and chapters, and received the Diplomate in Behavioral Psychology from the American Board of Professional Psychology. In collaboration with computer scientists at Georgia Tech, she has pioneered the application of virtual reality to the treatment of psychological disorders. Dr. Rothbaum has co-authored with Dr. Edna Foa, *Treating the Trauma of Rape: A Cognitive-Behavioral Therapy for PTSD* for practitioners treating PTSD.

EDNA B. FOA, PHD, Professor at the University of Pennsylvania, Director of the Center for the Treatment and Study of Anxiety, is an internationally renowned authority on the psychopathology and treatment of anxiety. Her research aiming at delineating etiological frameworks and targeted treatment has been highly influential and she is currently one of the leading experts in the areas of posttraumatic stress disorder. The program she has developed for rape survivors is considered to be the most effective therapy for post-trauma sequela. She has published several books and over 200 articles and book chapters, has lectured extensively around the world, and was the chair of the PTSD work group of the DSM-IV. Dr. Foa is the recipient of numerous awards and honors, including the Distinguished Scientist Award from the Scientific section of the American Psychological Association, the First Annual Outstanding Research Contribution Award from the Association for the Advancement of Behavior Therapy, the Distinguished Scientific Contributions to Clinical Psychology Award from the American Psychological Association and the Lifetime Achievement Award from the International Society for Traumatic Stress Studies.

Acknowledgments

We have so many people to acknowledge who have helped in some way bring this book about. We would like to thank the staff at the Violence and Traumatic Stress Program at the National Institute of Mental Health who have supported our work since 1986. It was then, in 1986, that we went to the Medical University of South Carolina in Charleston where we learned Stress Inoculation Training (SIT) from Dean Kilpatrick, PhD and Connie Best, PhD and their colleagues. Their pioneering work, along with Lois Veronen, PhD, really helped set the stage for our work.

This book is based in part on works of our colleagues and particularly the treatment manuals for our studies. At the Center for the Treatment and Study of Anxiety at the Medical College of Pennsylvania, our colleagues included Blanche Freund, Constance Dancu, Elizabeth Hembre, David Riggs, Michael Kozak, Lisa Jaycox, Elizabeth Meadows, Lori Zoellner, Norah Feeney, and Gordon Street. We thank David Clark for his help on the cognitive components of these manuals. More recently, we would like to thank Sheila Berry, who typed the final manuscript and worked on the references.

At The Trauma and Anxiety Recovery Program at Emory University School of Medicine, we would like to thank Barbara's colleagues for supporting her work there, including this book. They include Charles B. Nemeroff, MD, PhD, Philip T. Ninan, MD, Millie Astin, PhD, Trish Haugaard, and Bettina Knight, RN.

We would also like to thank the various individuals at The Psychological Corporation for their efforts and contributions. As Project Director, Sandra Prince-Embury, PhD, has coordinated the development of the Client Workbook and contributed significantly to the expression of the treatment in a form that is accessible to clients. Appreciation is also extended to those persons whose diligent and meticulous efforts were essential in preparing the Client Workbook. Among these individuals are Anthony Weyer MA, Research Assistant and Marian Zahora, Designer. Special appreciation is extended to Joanne Lenke, PhD, President; Aurelio Prifitera, PhD, Vice President and Director of the Psychological Measurement Group; and Larry Weiss, PhD, Director of the Behavioral Health Care and Personality Group.

Of course, our families deserve recognition for sacrificing their time with us for this work. John, Alex, and Jake Rothbaum and Faye, Sanford, Judy, Nathan, and Billy Olasov were never ending in their support and encouragement. Charles Kahn, Yael, and Michelle Foa endured an absentee wife and mother with only minimal complaints.

Most of all, we would like to thank the survivors we have worked with over the years who have allowed us to glimpse their personal nightmares of posttraumatic stress disorder. Through them, we learned, we gathered data, we tested techniques, and we grew as therapists, as scientists, and as people. We appreciate your courage and your willingness to share. Thank you.

Barbara O. Rothbaum
Atlanta, Georgia
December, 1998

Edna B. Foa
Philadelphia, Pennsylvania
December, 1998

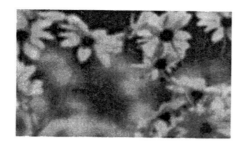

Introduction

Many of the emotional problems following a trauma are best described by a syndrome called Posttraumatic Stress Disorder (PTSD). The trauma is defined as a situation involving actual or threatened injury or death, and the survivor feels helpless, horrified, or terrified during the experience. Such traumatic life events, especially sexual and criminal assault, are unfortunately extremely common. It has been estimated that approximately one quarter of trauma survivors suffer from PTSD at some point in their lives. Women appear to be more likely than men to develop PTSD following trauma.

The magnitude of the problem can best be estimated from an excellent study in 1993 by Resnick and her colleagues that we will discuss in greater detail in Chapter 2. These researchers estimated that there are about 1.5 million adult female rape survivors who suffer from this disorder *right now*. They also calculated that about 4.5 million women in the U.S. are suffering from PTSD as you read this workbook. This makes PTSD an immense public health problem.

Not only is PTSD in general a monumental problem, but this is an ever growing problem as more women are being assaulted every hour. In our work as clinicians, we aim to help alleviate some of the suffering associated with these assaults. To this end, we have written this workbook for people actually suffering from PTSD or related problems. We have also written a book for professionals to teach them a treatment program that has been effective called *Treating the Trauma of Rape: Cognitive-Behavioral Therapy for PTSD*. The client workbook you are now reading is intended as a guide to help clients understand their treatment and practice helpful techniques that they will learn from their therapist, who may be using the related book for therapists. For those of you who are unfamiliar with the term "cognitive-behavioral" therapy, a very simple definition is a therapy that works through helping us be more aware of the power of our thoughts and to better observe and direct our own behavior.

In writing this book, we aim to address two goals. First, we want to present information about PTSD and related problems in language understandable to nonprofessionals. This information will include a review of the studies on posttrauma problems and on the effectiveness of different treatments. We will also describe why some survivors develop PTSD and others do not.

The second goal of the book is to provide a detailed client workbook for the treatment of trauma-related problems, especially PTSD, to assist clients working with a therapist. We are aware of the fact that people have different problems and different needs. What works for one person may not work for another. Therefore, we will describe several different treatment techniques. This book is organized around the different cognitive-behavioral techniques that have been studied and proven effective with women sufferers of PTSD following an assault. If you are in therapy, your therapist can discuss them with you and together you will decide which is the right program for you.

Throughout the book we will focus mainly on women who have been sexually assaulted and as a result developed chronic symptoms of PTSD, which have disturbed their daily functioning and cause them emotional distress. Most of the examples that we will use to demonstrate the cognitive-behavioral techniques are drawn from our experience in treating rape survivors. However, the cognitive-behavioral procedures outlined here have been as successful in helping women who have been sexually abused in childhood and adult female survivors of nonsexual assault, like aggravated assault and robbery. Other survivors of trauma such as natural disasters and car accidents were also helped by this cognitive-behavioral treatment. In addition, many of the cognitive-behavioral techniques described have been useful in the treatment of other anxiety disorders.

The book is divided into 5 sections. Section I focuses on what happens following an assault and contains 3 chapters. In Chapter 1 we describe the clinical picture of what happens following an assault using case examples. In Chapter 2 we will discuss the formal diagnosis of PTSD and the frequency of PTSD following different traumas. In Chapter 3 we discuss other problems that often occur after traumas.

Section II is an introduction to the cognitive-behavioral programs that are described in this book. It contains 4 chapters. Chapter 4 describes the various common reactions to assault, and offers questions for the reader to consider. In Chapter 5 we help you decide if you have PTSD by providing more specific questions. In Chapter 6 we review the studies of the different treatments of PTSD, including psychological and medication treatments. Chapter 7 introduces the treatment program and rationale that will help your therapist and you to decide what treatment (if any) is most appropriate for you.

Section III, which contains 3 chapters, is devoted to describing techniques called "exposure techniques" that have been shown to be effective for reducing PTSD. Chapter 8 teaches you how to relax. Chapter 9 deals with helping you confront actual situations that frighten you, and Chapter 10 helps you to deal with the traumatic memory of frightening events.

Section IV contains 3 chapters that focus on stress management techniques. Chapter 11 teaches you cognitive restructuring, a method used in cognitive therapy to help you examine your thinking to make sure you are thinking *rationally*. Chapter 12 discusses "thought-stopping," another cognitive therapy approach, to help stop obsessive thinking and preparing for a stressor to correct any negative self-talk, and Chapter 13 discusses covert modeling and role-play.

Section V has 2 chapters that discuss putting the treatment program all together. In Chapter 14 we discuss some common problems, and in Chapter 15 we help you plan your road for the future.

The book is written for those of you who are survivors of life's worst moments, and who are trying to overcome your devastating experiences. It is intended as a guide to help you in your journey to recapture your life and your old self. We have faith that it can happen, and your reading this book and working with a therapist is an excellent first step. We wish you luck, courage, strength, and peace of mind in your journey.

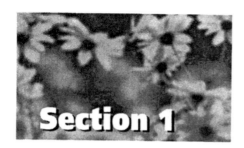

Section 1

After the Assault

Overview of PTSD and Other Reactions

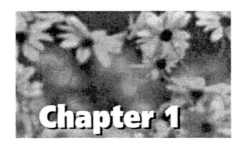

Chapter 1

Case Descriptions

It seems a good way to start this self-help guide about how to overcome post-rape difficulties by sharing with the reader an account of reactions to rape, as presented in our book for professionals (Foa & Rothbaum, 1998): the rape survivor's own report of the rape and how she reacted to being raped. This story describes clearly and powerfully the symptoms of posttraumatic stress disorder following sexual assault. Below is a powerful statement by Sarah, the survivor. This is followed by some reports from Sarah's father illustrating how the family may also be profoundly impacted by the event.

Sarah

Sarah's story about when the rape took place

It was in the summer when I was 16. I was babysitting that summer and was having a pretty good time until Wednesday of that week and then my life was shattered and all hell broke loose. On that Wednesday I decided to go for a walk and get away from things because I needed some peace and quiet. I was staying at a beach house a couple of hours from home with my next door neighbors and their two daughters. I went out of my bedroom door and went down to the beach to collect my thoughts. Being a babysitter for two active girls, I didn't have much time to do so. All of a sudden a man approached me from out of the blue. My back was to him and I didn't realize his presence until I felt his eyes from behind me and I flipped around unaware of any danger. As I turned around I had to squint my eyes because the outside light of the beach house was in my eyes. So, he could see me but I could only make out a figure of a man. From what I can remember, he was wearing all black and had a scent of cheap cologne. I have not smelled it since, and I hope I will never have to . . . anyway, I didn't realize I was in any danger until he came closer to me, and I could feel his eyes staring straight at me. I was only 16 and I lived in the suburbs. I was pretty oblivious to danger and in a way I trusted him because I just trusted people.

Now, I trust no one unless I know them well enough to my satisfaction. He came closer to me and I could feel his breath. He was taller than me but then again, everyone was tall to me. All I saw was black until I looked around and saw, for the first time, a long knife in his left hand. It sparkled in the light and again, I could only make out a manly figure. I never saw his face because he was wearing a ski mask, but I could feel his eyes and that is enough for me. I am so glad I didn't see his face or my nightmares would probably be worse and more vivid than they are now. He pulled me out of the light and pushed me back toward some bushes. He told me I could either run and he would kill me, or I could stay and we could have a lot of fun. I still remember his voice. I can't describe it but it is permanently in my mind. I didn't answer. He held the knife up to my throat and looked at me. Then, he pushed me down to the ground on my back and ripped off my shorts and underpants. It took him a little to get ready himself. Then, he forced himself down on me. He was very heavy and strong. I felt that, so I didn't struggle, and I think that was smart. He did have a knife and who knows what else. Then I felt the pain from the lower end of my body and then that's when I knew what this horrible man was doing to me. He was raping me. Not only raping up my insides but my trust, my honesty, my cleanliness, my pride, my sleep, my friends, my family, my happiness, and most of all, my life.

I just lay there not doing anything but thinking, "What am I going to tell my family?" I don't recall how long this went on but I do recall the pain and the powerlessness. Then, a wet feeling. Then he got up and said, "Thanks." That's all he said and he left and went on his way to rape another, or home to his wife and kids, or back to a house out on the street. I don't know and don't care at all. After he left, I just sat there and tried to think up some sort of reasonable solution of what to do. So I gathered my clothes and headed back to the house. Not as I had before when I had no violent thoughts in my mind. I have never really walked the same way since. Now, always with distrust of the situation and myself.

Sarah after the rape . . .

I safely got back in the house, and immediately went to the shower. Now I was sobbing lightly but not wanting to let the people upstairs hear me. They were eating dinner and having a good time while I was being ripped apart. When I got in the shower, the first thing I grabbed for was the soap. I washed every part of my body and now I was crying. Now I was scared of everything I had trusted before tonight. Finally, after washing myself very thoroughly as best I could, I got out. I didn't want to because I still was not clean and I wanted to stay in there until I was. But I got out, dried off, and headed to bed. I did not sleep for at least one month. The most I got was 30-minute spurts and then I was wide awake waiting for him to come back and do it all over again. Well, I managed to get through the week, I don't know how. That will always amaze me. But I did go home and started my period so that was some sort of comfort to me.

Sarah described how difficult it was to share with her family what had happened

. . . It was toward the end of my 11th grade year, at the end-of-the-year church banquet for the youth. My brother, Billy, and I were coming home, and we dropped off one of his friends, now one of my friends, and we started back home. Having seen all those slides of the past year's mission project brought back sudden memories. I just felt so close to him that I told him everything. All he said during that time was "yeah." He was upset, I could tell. He was angry, but not at me. I knew that. He was angry at the life I had. When we got home, we hugged and I made him promise not to tell anyone, especially mom and dad. He kept that promise as long as possible and as long as I needed him to keep it. Well, one of the girls with whom I shared what happened in the previous summer's mission project told her mother who couldn't keep it silent any longer. She made an appointment with my dad one or two days after my brother Billy's college graduation—well, then everything in my perfectly planned life fell apart, and my mom found out, and then, my older brother found out. Then I realized that everyone knew. That Monday night I had to tell my family everything. That was no picnic for me but the only good thing was that Billy was right there beside me during the whole time. He was on my side. I am really glad I told him before everybody else found out, because I don't think he and I would be as close as we are right now. That summer, after I told my family, was very hard for me because I thought they believed I was unclean, and of course, raped. Well, I got help and love.

The father's reaction to learning about the rape and description of Sarah's reaction

> All of a sudden, the change in Sarah's behavior in the past two years made sense. I began to understand why this dynamic, strong-willed, but kind person had become contentious, aggressive, demanding, and hostile at the smallest provocation. I realized why, all of a sudden, Sarah had refused to go to school. At the time, we probed and questioned. I spoke with several of her friends, searching for information that would help me understand the dramatic changes in Sarah, but we received no answer. Sarah persistently refused to discuss any problems, and her outbursts following our attempts at communicating with her rendered our inquiries extremely painful. Her patterns at school paralleled the home demeanor. We were informed by teachers that Sarah was argumentative, hostile and disruptive, insensitive to the needs of her peers, and inconsiderate of her teachers. Sarah's conflicts with the gym faculty were particularly severe. She refused to participate in gym, resisted wearing the required garb, frequently reporting that her equipment had been stolen from her locker, and promptly "lost" whatever new gym equipment we purchased. It seemed to us that Sarah was intentionally marginalizing herself at school. We had no idea of any antecedent cause. Surprisingly, she passed all her academic subjects that year.
>
> Sarah became an enraged, hostile and defiant 17-year-old, oblivious, from our perspective, to the consequences of her actions. She was particularly verbally brutal to her mother. Sarah verbally attacked her over trivial issues, and frequently questioned her love and caring. Nothing that either of us did during those two years tempered the emotional difficulties that invaded our home. The crisis only intensified. Later, we found out Sarah contemplated suicide in that first year, so, retrospectively, I am relieved that she turned her rage towards us as she did. While Sarah's behavior has become compre-hensible now, this understanding was accompanied with excruciating pain.

Sarah's father writes about what he learned from his own experience about PTSD and its treatment

> Treatment must facilitate the reintegration of the traumatic event and its impact into the ongoing psychological life of the individual; that is, the event must become an "object" to be

scrutinized and understood as something that has happened to the person. It means being able to tolerate imaging the entire trauma event and its sequelae, and experiencing the concomitant pain without turning away. The trauma event must become, over time, simply a life event within a sequence of other remembered life events. These trauma memories must become devoid of the emotional arousal and reflexive activity that characterize the original disorder.

To achieve these goals, our family now understands that therapy must guide the survivor in a gentle but consistently directed manner, to reconstruct verbally all components of the trauma event. This must be done repetitively, until all parts of the trauma can be constructed into *the story*. Once the story can be told in its entirety, the emotional upset can be gradually extinguished in the safety of the therapy environment. Reintegration of the Self will accompany this reconstruction process.

The goal of this workbook is to teach the reader how to "reconstruct verbally all components of the trauma event" so that PTSD symptoms and their damaging effects will diminish.

Sarah and her father's reactions are an exceptional example of how a traumatic event demolishes the survivors' positive views about the world and themselves. It portrays how survivors' feelings and ideas about the essence of their existence suddenly change, leaving them estranged from themselves and from others, helpless, and hopeless, in the midst of a seemingly hostile world.

The rest of this chapter relates the story of other survivors to further illustrate the devastating impact of rape.

Stephanie

Stephanie, who was raped during a date with a friend, relates a similar story

I assumed he wouldn't hurt me because I hadn't done anything to deserve to be hurt. I didn't know there were people who would hurt you anyway. I didn't know that the person I was had power. Afterwards, I felt like I'd been broken, like a bottle. At a party the next night with my co-workers, I felt like shouting, "Can't you see I'm different? Can't you see I'm not the same person I was last week? Why aren't you saying anything about it? I know you can see I'm different."

Toward the end of therapy, Stephanie had recovered her self

It's clear to me that in some ways I'm more than one person. When these things happened to me, this part of me almost died, she went somewhere and waited for me to come out and live this life I've always wanted to live. I would like to enjoy my body again. I was not born to make other people feel better or to let these men feel more like men by doing disgusting things to my body. That is not why I was born. My body is mine, it's okay to ask for what I want. The dark days are over. It feels good to realize that the hardest part of my life is over. I'm not afraid of the hard stuff ahead. I can feel happiness.

Naomi

Naomi's story of early and prolonged abuse

Naomi's story is different from those of Sarah or Stephanie as she was sexually and physically abused during her childhood and adolescence by her mother's boyfriend, Darryl. It all began when Darryl moved in to live with Naomi and her mother when Naomi was 8 years old. At first, he used to fondle her inappropriately, especially when her mother worked nights and he was drunk. With time Darryl became increasingly abusive both sexually and emotionally, threatening to hurt her more if she ever told anyone about the abuse. He explained that he was doing her a favor, getting her ready to deal with other men. Sexual penetration started when Naomi was 10 years old and continued until she was 15. Being the oldest child, and aware of how hard her mother's life was trying to raise her and her younger sister, Naomi did not want to burden her with her situation.

I didn't know what to do. I couldn't tell anybody, I couldn't stop it, I was stuck. At first, when I would try to fight him, he hurt me bad, so I didn't try anymore. Then I figured out a way to leave my body. In my mind, I would float out of my body, go out the door, and go out the apartment. I started walking around the neighborhood in my mind. It was dark, at night, when he was doing it to me, and after a while I figured out how to make it daytime in my head. I would go to this park, not a real one, but a wonderful one I made up, and I would spend my time there until he left. Sometimes, he would want me to talk to him, to tell him I liked it or something, and then that would ruin my visit to the park, and I'd cry myself to sleep.

Naomi ran away from home when she was 15 years old and had a difficult life on the streets. She often exchanged sex for drugs, food, or lodging, and was physically and sexually abused.

> It's like it didn't matter when someone beat up on me or raped me; it's like I expected them to, almost deserved it for trying to get away. Sometimes I would try to go to the park in my head, sometimes I was so messed up I was out of it, and sometimes I would get wasted as soon as it was over. This is what I thought life was.

For years Naomi suffered from depression, alcohol and drug dependence, dissociation, and PTSD. She sought treatment when she was 32 years old following a rape by an acquaintance.

The stories reported in this chapter are powerful and thought provoking. If you are also a survivor of sexual assault, these stories may have triggered thoughts and feelings related to your own experience. Take a minute to think about and maybe write down these thoughts and feelings. The following chapters provide more explanations of trauma and post-traumatic stress symptoms.

Additional Reading

Foa, E. B., & Rothbaum, B. O. (1998). *Treating the trauma of rape: Cognitive-behavioral therapy for PTSD.* New York: Guilford Press.

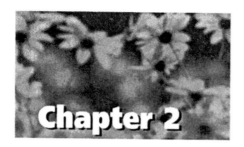

Chapter 2

Posttraumatic Stress Disorder Following Assault

What is a Trauma?

A trauma is an extremely painful emotional experience that poses threat of injury or death and makes the person feel terrified and helpless. Thus, trauma includes both objective aspects of threat and subjective aspects of extreme negative emotions. Accordingly, a car accident may or may not be traumatic. If it severely disrupts the person's life and causes substantial emotional distress, we call it a trauma. If it causes some transitory fear and does not leave much of a mark on the person, we wouldn't call it a trauma. Therefore, a trauma is in part defined by what is traumatic for you. Also, a traumatic experience does not necessarily mean that you yourself have been threatened. One can become traumatized by witnessing someone else being killed or injured, or even by hearing about a disaster that happened to significant others. For example, witnessing someone burning in a fire is traumatic as is the visit of army representatives to notify a mother that her son was killed in the war.

If you are in therapy, it is important to let your therapist know about any of these events you have experienced, so that he/she can evaluate if you need to work on your trauma.

What is Posttraumatic Stress Disorder?

The definition of Posttraumatic Stress Disorder (PTSD) has been determined by experts in the field and is included in *The Diagnostic and Statistical Manual (DSM) of Mental Disorders* with all other psychiatric disorders. The DSM describes PTSD as an Anxiety Disorder characterized by persisting symptoms of reexperiencing (e.g., nightmares, flashbacks), avoidance and numbing (e.g., avoidance of reminders, decreased interest in activities), and arousal (e.g., difficulty sleeping, exaggerated startle). As we noted above, the most recent version of the DSM, the *DSM-IV* (APA, 1994), has defined the traumatic experience as an objectively dangerous event that has caused strong fear reactions and a sense of helplessness.

Table 2.1 is a description of the PTSD symptoms according to the *DSM-IV*. Please check all the symptoms that you are currently experiencing.

Table 2.1. **PTSD Symptoms**

I. Reexperiencing the traumatic event:

   1. thoughts, images, or ideas about the trauma that keep coming back and are unwanted and cause distress

   2. nightmares or bad dreams about the trauma or that seem related to it

   3. flashbacks of the traumatic event, as if it were happening again

   4. extreme emotional distress when you are reminded of the traumatic event

   5. extreme bodily reactions when you are reminded of the traumatic event (for example, heart races, get sweaty, tense up)

II. Continual avoidance of reminders of the traumatic event and/or emotional numbing:

   1. avoid thinking about, talking about, or feelings associated with the trauma

   2. avoid situations, activities, places, or people that remind you of the traumatic event

   3. can't remember *important* parts of what happened

   4. large decrease in interest or time spent in activities that were important to you

   5. feeling of being cut off from other people and inability to connect to them

   6. emotional numbing; being unable to experience the whole range of emotions that you used to feel

   7. feeling that your life will be cut short; not expecting to live as long as you had thought

III. Indications of increased arousal:

1. persistent problems falling or staying asleep

2. extreme irritability or outbursts of anger

3. persistent difficulty concentrating

4. extreme alertness to your environment, checking the situation all around you, being hypervigilant

5. extremely jumpy, startle very easily

If you have experienced a traumatic event and you suffer from several of these symptoms you are likely to suffer from PTSD. In Chapter 5 we will guide you in deciding if you indeed have PTSD. In this chapter we review what research has taught us about PTSD reactions following trauma.

Trauma reactions have been recognized for more than a century. In that time, they have been called by many different names, such as "war neurosis," and "rape trauma syndrome." The duration of PTSD symptoms can vary greatly from person to person. Some survivors who have experienced traumatic events may have apparently few or no long-lasting effects, whereas others may have problems even years after the trauma.

The Symptoms of Posttraumatic Stress Disorder Following an Assault

Experts have noticed that criminal victimization produces a variety of psychological disturbances including anxiety, depression, intrusive thoughts and images of the assault, and sleep disturbances such as nightmares and insomnia. Rape survivors report that thoughts and images of the assault come to their mind automatically. These thoughts are so distressing that survivors put a lot of effort in trying to push them away. They also report substantial sleeping problems such as difficulty falling to sleep and waking up in the middle of the night. Fearing the recurrence of nightmares, survivors often delay going to bed until they are exhausted. Difficulty concentrating is another common symptom in assault survivors. Thus, the postassault psychological problems can be best described as PTSD.

The Course of PTSD in Trauma Survivors

After a major trauma, most people will experience psychological problems. However, most will recover over time on their own. Therefore, it is important to distinguish between normal reactions to trauma and chronic reactions that require treatment. Studies (see the Additional Reading section for more information) have indicated that an assault is a traumatic event and almost everyone who experiences an assault, and particularly sexual assault, will experience significant PTSD symptoms immediately following it. If a person continues to improve after an assault, he/she may not need to seek treatment. But, if they are stuck in a bad place, and things do not seem to be getting any better, they may want to get help sooner rather than later.

The Prevalence of PTSD Among Trauma Survivors

Several experts studied women who had been sexually assaulted and assessed their PTSD retrospectively, that is, looking backwards from the time of the assessment back to the rape and asking them to recall symptoms they may have experienced. These studies have not found as high a rate of PTSD as in studies using a prospective method that assesses symptoms as the person is experiencing them.

The rate of trauma and PTSD were assessed in a group of 4008 American women in 1993 using telephone interviews. Resnick and her colleagues used the results of this study to estimate the number of women in the United States who had experienced the different types of traumas based on the 1989 US Bureau of the Census Estimate of the population of US adult women. According to this estimation, approximately 12,151,084 American women have experienced a completed rape, and about 4 million have suffered from PTSD as a result of rape. Moreover, about two-thirds of adult American women have experienced a significant trauma, with a large percentage of them having PTSD at some point after the trauma. Women who had experienced a criminal trauma were three times as likely to have PTSD at the time of the interview than women who experienced other traumas such as natural disasters. The implications of this important study for health in general and mental health in particular are enormous as it suggests that criminal victimization and the resultant PTSD are a serious health problem for American women.

It is clear from the studies of rape and crime survivors that a high rate of PTSD immediately after the assault which decreases gradually over time is common, but some women, especially those who were raped, develop chronic PTSD that can last for many years.

Numbing, Dissociation, and PTSD

Dissociative experiences during and immediately after a trauma are common. Dissociative symptoms during or shortly after a trauma seem to be a strong predictor of developing PTSD. Dissociative symptoms are common in Acute Stress Disorder, and numbing symptoms are present in PTSD. Therefore, we will now discuss what "dissociation" means and how it is related to "numbing."

Many experts have focused on the fear and anxiety aspects of PTSD, but in addition to these reactions, other commonly observed reactions are emotional numbing and cognitive avoidance of situations, objects, or memories that are trauma reminders. These reactions, referred to as dissociation, denial, or numbing, include a decreased awareness of one's emotions or thoughts that some experts think serves as a means of reducing emotional and physical pain and are commonly exhibited by persons who have experienced trauma. Dissociative symptoms include amnesia, feelings of depersonalization, out-of-body experiences, dream-like recall of events, feelings of estrangement, flashbacks, and abreaction. A second related concept, denial, includes avoidance of reminders of the trauma without changes in perception or memory problems. Yet another term is "numbing," that describes the periodic lack of emotional expression that trauma survivors experience in circumstances that call for emotional reaction.

The seven symptoms that make up the avoidance/numbing cluster of DSM-IV PTSD diagnosis include: cognitive and behavioral avoidance of trauma reminders, memory loss, loss of interest in activities, feeling cut off from others, restricted emotions/feeling emotionally numb, and sense of a foreshortened future (e.g., thinking you may not live as long as you had thought; APA, 1994).

Conclusion

Almost all survivors of severe trauma such as rape will suffer from PTSD symptoms and these symptoms will continue for days or weeks. After a traumatic experience, one of three results is likely to occur over time. First, most survivors show reduction of the symptoms in the long run. Although they will never forget the trauma and most likely will be mildly distressed when remembering it, they resume their normal lives. Second, some survivors will develop chronic but limited symptoms that can be diagnosed as a specific phobia, like fearing and avoiding dogs after being attacked by a dog. Third, about 10% to 15% of survivors of severe traumas will develop full chronic PTSD, which includes flashbacks, nightmares and numbing or dissociative symptoms, in addition to specific fears.

Additional Reading

American Psychiatric Association (APA). (1994). *Diagnostic and statistical manual of mental disorders.* (4th ed.). Washington, DC: Author.

Resnick, H. S., Kilpatrick, D. G., Dansky, B. S., Saunders, B. E., & Best, C. L. (1993). Prevalence of civilian trauma and posttraumatic stress disorder in a representative national sample of women. *Journal of Consulting and Clinical Psychology, 61*(6), 984-991.

Riggs, D. S., Rothbaum, B. O., & Foa, E. B. (1995). A prospective examination of symptoms of posttraumatic stress disorder in survivors of non-sexual assault. *Journal of Interpersonal Violence, 10*(2), 201-214.

Rothbaum, B. O., Foa, E. B., Riggs, D. S., Murdock, T., & Walsh, W. (1992). A prospective examination of post-traumatic stress disorder in rape victims. *Journal of Traumatic Stress, 5*(3), 455-475.

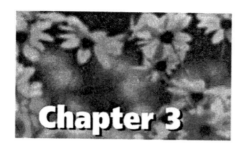

Chapter 3

Other Reactions to Assault

Posttraumatic stress disorder describes the most typical reactions to assault and other traumas. However, other reactions are also common. Many of these other problems also improve with the treatment for PTSD that we will describe in this book, but some trauma-related reactions may require special attention. This review is not meant to be complete but does focus on other reactions that are common after an assault.

Emotional Reactions

Depression

Depression is also a common reaction to rape. Research suggests that depression experienced by survivors is not as long lasting as anxiety, although research findings are mixed on this topic. Some studies showed that about half of rape survivors were depressed for a long time after the assault, even up to an average of 22 years postassault. It has also been found that women who were raped more than one time were more likely to suffer from depression. These findings suggest that for a considerable number of survivors, particularly survivors of multiple assaults, depression will be a long lasting problem.

A reaction related to depression is contemplating suicide. Studies estimate the number of survivors who have considered suicide following their assault range from 2.9% to 50%. Clearly, suicidal thoughts occur to many survivors. If you are seriously considering suicide, we urge you to talk to your therapist or other mental health professional. You will not be considered "crazy"; all mental health professionals who work with rape survivors know that this is common. Please seek professional help.

Anger

As we may expect, anger is definitely a common reaction among survivors of assault. It is understandable that anytime we are treated wrongly, and most definitely when we are assaulted, anger is a natural and justified reaction. However, there is some evidence that holding on to rage can interfere with recovery. We may conclude that although anger is a natural reaction to assault, working through the anger is a necessary part of healing. If you feel that your anger interferes with your daily functioning and with your recovery, you may need to pay particular attention to this issue.

Shame

Many rape survivors report feeling a great deal of shame. This may interfere with their willingness to talk about what happened to them. Although shame is very common following rape, it is important to work on this in therapy.

Dissociation

In Chapter 2 we have discussed dissociation as it relates to PTSD. Here we want to discuss the symptoms and experience of dissociation. The DSM-IV (APA, 1994) describes Dissociation as a "disruption in the usually integrated functions of consciousness, memory, identity, or perception of the environment." The experience of dissociation in everyday life can occur in ways that may be barely noticeable. For example, you may realize that you have not been paying attention to where you were driving while you were travelling on a route that was very familiar to you, like being on "automatic pilot." The most extreme form of dissociation is Multiple Personality Disorder (MPD), now known as Dissociative Identity Disorder (DID). It is described in the DSM–III–R as "the presence of two or more distinct identities or personality states." A whole range of dissociative experiences lies in between these two extremes.

Extreme forms of dissociation such as dissociative identity disorder are now understood to be the result of traumatic experience. In a study of 100 people with multiple personality disorder (MPD), 97% were found to have had a major childhood trauma, such as incest, physical abuse, physical and sexual abuse combined, extreme neglect, and witnessing a violent death. See the 1986 study by Putnam and colleagues for additional reading. It is now understood that in these instances dissociation allows the person to emotionally remove himself/herself from a traumatic event when physical escape seems impossible. It is not uncommon for rape survivors to report that during the assault they tried to emotionally leave their bodies.

Social Problems

Several studies have found evidence that the experience of rape may also affect social functioning in many ways. Negative impact on social functioning may be manifested in increased marital and family problems or decreased range or time spent in engaging in social activities. Problems in social functioning may be caused by fears of strangers, of going out with new people, and of people walking behind them, so that survivors may avoid many safe social and leisure activities. Conflicting findings in some studies suggest that the negative impact of rape on marriage and family life may relate to other factors, so these effects may occur more for some survivors than for others.

Sexual Problems

As we would expect, sexual problems following rape are common. Fear of sex and decreased sexual arousal or desire are the most common problems. This reaction can impact on the frequency of sexual behavior, especially soon after the assault. Two weeks after the assault, the majority of survivors said they had sex less frequently since the assault. By four weeks postassault, almost half noted they avoided sex completely. However for many, this effect on frequency grew less over time. The frequency of sex had improved by four months and had nearly returned to preassault levels by one year after the assault.

However, negative effects on sexuality can persist for many after the rape. Sexually induced flashbacks were reported by many survivors one year after the assault. In addition, some survivors experienced less sexual satisfaction one and a half years postassault than nonvictims.

Trust

Many survivors report difficulty trusting others following an assault. Most of us grow up with a belief in human kindness, but the assault shatters this assumption with the intentionally cruel act of one human against another. It takes a long time to work on restoring this lost trust. Survivors work on relearning who to trust and who not to trust. It is often very difficult for survivors to trust their therapists. Also, they may not trust themselves anymore. These are all issues to be worked on in therapy and in life following an assault.

Table 3.1 contains a summary of the common reactions to assault we discuss in this chapter with some references to research articles. If you are interested in reading more on any of these topics, complete references are provided in the Additional Readings section.

Table 3.1.	Common Reactions to Assault	

Reaction	Sample	Readings
Depression	Rape Survivors	Frank & Stewart, 1984; Nadelson, Notman, Zackson, & Gornick, 1982
Anger	Rape Survivors	Riggs, Dancu, Gershuny, Greenberg, & Foa, 1992
Dissociation	Sexual Assault Survivors	Bernstein & Putnam, 1986; Dancu, Rothbaum, Riggs, & Foa, 1990; Putnam et al., 1986
Social Maladjustment	Rape Survivors	Nadelson et al., 1982
Work Difficulties	Rape Survivors	Kilpatrick, Veronen, & Resick, 1979; Resick, Calhoun, Atkeson, & Ellis, 1981
Sexual Problems	Rape Survivors	Becker, Skinner, Abel, & Treacy, 1982; Nadelson et al., 1982

In reality, a traumatic experience causes many different reactions and difficulties. As described above, these reactions include PTSD symptoms, general anxiety, depression, anger, shame, mistrust, dissociation, social problems and sexual difficulties. Many of these reactions subside over time but some linger for a long time. Although the treatment described in this client workbook addresses your PTSD symptoms specifically, we have found that when PTSD is treated successfully, many of the other reactions improve as well.

In Chapters 2 and 3 we have summarized the results of many studies about common reactions to rape and other trauma survivors. We hope that reading about these common reactions will help you understand your own reactions. You may not experience many of the reactions that we described. Not all survivors do. Or, you may be experiencing some common reactions that we have not discussed yet. The studies present how people react on the average, and that means that there are many individual differences. These chapters are meant as a guide to understanding your reactions.

Additional Reading

American Psychiatric Association (APA). (1994). *Diagnostic and statistical manual of mental disorders*. (4th ed.). Washington, DC: Author.

Putnam, F. W., Guroff, J. J., Silberman, E. K., Barban, L., & Post, R. M. (1986). The clinical phenomenology of multiple personality disorder: Review of 100 recent cases. *Journal of Clinical Psychiatry, 47*(6), 285-293.

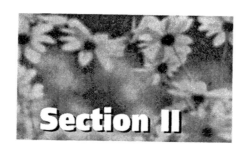

Section II

Assessing Personal Reactions

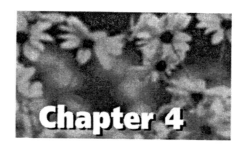

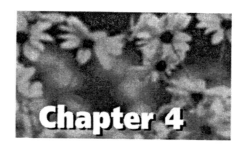

Chapter 4

Common Reactions to Assault

In this chapter, we discuss again some of the common reactions to assault. Throughout this discussion, we urge you to think about your own reactions and how your own experiences are similar or different from what we describe. If you are currently in therapy, it is helpful to discuss this with your therapist as well. You may find it helpful to write down your thoughts and observations about yourself. The act of writing down some of the reactions and problems will help you see more clearly what you are experiencing as a result of the assault, and this in turn will help you and your therapist design your treatment program. You may identify a notebook or diary that you can devote to this program.

This chapter may be shown to close friends and relatives so that they can understand more about what you are going through.

An assault is a severe trauma which produces an emotional shock, a great deal of distress and other types of common reactions. In later chapters we will discuss why some people continue to have difficulties long after the assault and will explain how the treatment will work to alleviate your distress. As previously discussed, some reactions are common to traumatic experiences, but each person responds in his or her own unique way. Also many changes in emotional reaction after a trauma are common. In fact, 95% of rape survivors have severe problems two weeks after the rape. About half of these women feel much better within three months after the rape. The other 50% of survivors recover more slowly, and many do not recover enough without help. Becoming more aware of the changes you've undergone since your assault is the first step toward recovery. The following are specific questions to help you more clearly understand your reaction if you have suffered an assault.

1. The principal reactions people experience after an assault are *fear* and *anxiety*.

   Do you find yourself frequently feeling fearful, tense or anxious?

   We have found that survivors experience feelings of anxiety when reminded of the assault. For many survivors it seems to come out of nowhere, unrelated to anything.

   One way to explore these feelings is to begin to notice whether you are more fearful at certain times than others. Are you more frightened in particular instances than others?

   The anxiety and fear experienced in a dangerous and life-threatening situation may last long after the assault had ended. This extended reaction exists because trauma can trigger emotional, physical and cognitive changes in you, because the way you perceive your surroundings and your views about personal safety have changed as a result of the traumatic event. Because these changes persist after the event, you may become anxious when you remember your assault. You may wonder about the times that anxiety appears to come from nowhere. This may occur because certain *triggers* and *cues* subtly bring to mind memories of the assault and you may start to feel afraid. These triggers may be certain times of the day, certain places, men approaching you, an argument with someone you care about, or a certain smell or noise. As you begin to pay more attention to the times you feel afraid, you can discover the triggers for your anxiety. In this way, you may learn that some of the out of the blue anxiety is really triggered by things that remind you of your assault.

   With the above explanation in mind, think of specific triggers that remind you of the assault and write them down now in your notebook.

   Typically, after an assault, fear and anxiety are experienced in a number of ways: (a) re-experiencing memories of the assault, (b) frequently feeling nervous, easily startled and jumpy, and (c) isolating yourself from others and not going places.

   Although it may be difficult at first, we want you to note the changes that you may be experiencing in your body, your feelings and your thoughts that have resulted from the assault/rape. Your observation of your own reactions is very important to your treatment.

2. In addition, assault survivors *re-experience* the traumatic event. If visual pictures of the assailant's face or some other aspect of the assault suddenly pops into your mind, you are re-experiencing the trauma, or having a flashback.

   If you are having flashbacks, what is this experience like for you? Please write this down in your notebook.

Some flashbacks may seem so real that you might believe that the assault is happening all over again. These flashbacks are intrusive and you probably feel that you don't have any control over what you are feeling, thinking, and experiencing during the day or at night. As mentioned previously, flashbacks are triggered by things in your surroundings, and often you might not recognize what triggers them.

Another common way that survivors re-experience the assault is through *nightmares* while sleeping.

Are you experiencing nightmares while you are asleep? When you wake up after having a nightmare, what physical reactions do you have?

Reexperiencing of the assault may also occur emotionally or cognitively (*unwanted thoughts*) without having a flashback or nightmare.

Have you been having upsetting thoughts and feelings about what happened to you?

3. Many assault survivors have *trouble concentrating* following their assault.

Trouble with concentrating may make reading difficult. Following a conversation, or remembering something that someone told you may also be more difficult than before. Have you experienced any of these difficulties yourself?

Trouble being able to concentrate, remember, and pay attention to what is going on around you makes it more difficult to function in your daily life. You may sometimes *feel that you are not in control of your mind or a feeling that you are going crazy*. It is important to remind yourself that these reactions will go away in time. Problems you have in trying to focus your attention on something may be the result of disturbing recollections of the trauma and accompanying emotional reactions. These symptoms occur because a traumatic experience is so shocking and so different from everyday experiences that you can't fit it into what you know about the world. Because of this, your brain is constantly reviewing the traumatic event to try and figure out what had happened and try to comprehend it all. This major undertaking may make it hard for your brain to concentrate on other tasks for long periods of time.

4. Another common reaction to assault is a heightened state of *arousal* (that is, feeling nervous or "wound-up"). Heightened arousal is displayed in increased agitation, feeling jittery, feeling *overly alert*, trembling, being *easily startled*, and having trouble sleeping.

Are you experiencing any of these reactions since the trauma? Are there times when you feel panic? What bodily changes occur during those times? Sweating? Heart beating really fast? Do you find yourself being especially on the lookout for signs of danger in your surroundings?

Are you very jumpy or on edge? Please write down in your notebook what you have been experiencing, when it occurs, and about how frequently.

If you are tense and jumpy all the time, you may also find yourself feeling more *irritable*. This is especially likely to occur if you are having problems sleeping.

Have you been feeling irritable or angry? Do you find that you are having angry outbursts or that you are more snappy than usual with people?

Many of the changes described above may result from fear. Animals and people have several potential reactions to being startled, assaulted, or threatened. One response to a threatening situation is to *freeze*. You may have seen a cat that is being approached by a dog crouch down and be very still because it is afraid. Another danger response is to *run away* or *flee*. A third response to a threat is to *fight*. Have you ever seen a cat puff up its fur, hiss, extend its claws, and swat at a threatening dog?

When a threat is encountered, a surge of adrenaline is needed to enable the body to respond by either fighting or running away. As a result of the assault, you may be more aware of the possibility of being in a dangerous situation, and you want to be prepared to deal with it. Your heightened arousal is your experience of your body being pumped up and able to quickly react to any sudden danger. It is true that a ready state helps when you are faced with actual danger, such as if you were in a burning building. However, remaining at that high level of alertness becomes very uncomfortable when it continues for a long time, even in safe situations.

5. It is common for survivors to avoid people, locations, or objects that bring up memories of the assault. This *avoidance* may be actual physical avoidance, as well as avoidance in thought or feeling. The most common is avoiding situations that remind you of the assault, such as the place where it happened. Often situations that are less directly related to the trauma are also avoided, such as going out in the evening if you were assaulted at night. This avoidance is a strategy to protect yourself from situations that you may feel have become dangerous, and thoughts and feelings that are overwhelming and upsetting.

   Ask yourself the following question: Are you unable to go certain places or do certain things as a result of the assault? Have you been making efforts to avoid thoughts or feelings associated with the assault? How do you do that? What kinds of things do you find yourself doing to try to forget what happened to you? Please write some of these down.

   You might find that you are not able to remember pertinent details of the assault because of a strong desire not to experience the emotions and thoughts that are associated with the assault. This may be a form of cognitive avoidance.

Do you find that there are missing periods of time or absent details when you recall what happened during the assault?

Emotional numbness is a common reaction you may have that is related to pushing away painful feelings and thoughts about the assault. This reaction occurs when conflicting emotions are present and you find it hard to feel love or kindness in conjunction with being afraid.

Do you notice feeling numb, empty, or removed from what is going on around you? Have you found that you no longer care about doing things that you used to enjoy? Do you feel detached and isolated from others following the assault? Please write down what types of situations trigger this numbing response.

6. Individuals who have survived an assault often feel *sadness* and *a sense of feeling down* or *depressed*. This sadness may also bring feelings of hopelessness and despair, frequent crying spells, and sometimes even thoughts of hurting yourself and suicide. A *loss of interest* in the people and activities that you once found enjoyable may result in a joyless life. It may seem that you are no longer able to have fun or enjoy anything. You may also feel that life isn't worth living and that plans you had made for the future do not seem important any longer. These feelings can lead to thoughts of wishing you were dead or doing something to hurt or kill yourself. Because the assault has changed so much of how you see the world and yourself, it is not surprising to feel sad and to grieve for what seems to have been lost following the assault.

Have you been feeling sad or depressed? Are you tearful? Are you feeling stuck or hopeless? Are you having any feelings or ideas that life is not worth living or that you would be better off dead?

7. You may have been threatened and made to do things that you did not want to do when you were assaulted. You were violated. You may have felt that you could *not control* your body, what you were feeling, and your well being and safety. You may be re-experiencing feelings of not having control and think that you are *"going crazy"* or *"losing it"* as a result.

Have you felt a loss of control after the assault? What is that like for you? Are you able to do anything that helps you to deal with these thoughts and emotions?

8. Survivors often have feelings of *guilt* and *shame*. These feelings may be related to something you did or did not do to survive the assault. It is common to second guess your reactions and blame yourself for what you did or did not do.

Are you blaming yourself for the assault? Do you feel that if you had or had not done something that you would not have been assaulted?

Are there any people that you are avoiding talking to or things that you are avoiding doing because you feel guilty or ashamed?

Many survivors feel ashamed if they were made to do something that they would not do in other situations. This feeling may result from a belief that if they had acted in another manner (offered less resistance or fought their way out of the situation), their assault would not have been so bad. If you have feelings of guilt for what happened during the assault, you are taking personal responsibility for what the attacker did to you. These feelings of guilt can lead to feelings of helplessness, depression, and negative thoughts about yourself. Blame can also come from society in general, people who are close to you, loved ones, relatives, and acquaintances because many times people place responsibility on the person who has been hurt and survived. The blame placed by others is often related to their difficulty in accepting the possibility of feeling helpless and the idea that others could inflict harm intentionally.

Has anyone blamed you for the assault? How do you feel about that? Would you blame your sister or your daughter if the same thing happened to her?

You must keep reminding yourself that being assaulted was not a result of anything you did or were responsible for. You did not ask to be treated badly or harmed by someone else. No one has the right to harm you, regardless of anything you did or did not do. Even if you feel you made a mistake in judgment, people make mistakes in judgment every day. In this case the "punishment" didn't fit the "crime." The only time someone has the right to hurt you is if you hurt them first and they are acting in self-defense, and that is not what happened here.

9. *Anger* is frequently reported by survivors of assault. The anger is mostly directed at the assailant for causing you physical injury, for violating you, for abusing you, or for stealing something of yours. You must also recognize that you may start to feel anger when you encounter people who bring back memories of the attacker or strangers. Many assault survivors also feel angry at God for allowing them to be assaulted, at the police for not doing enough afterwards, at the hospital staff for treating them insensitively, at society for creating an atmosphere that allows this to happen, and at friends and family for not understanding. Sometimes our anger about the assault is so intense that it gets expressed across many people and circumstances in a way that we don't fully understand.

Have you been feeling particularly angry or aggressive? Is feeling this way a change from how you felt previous to the assault? What do you think about having these feelings and what their impact on yourself and others is?

You may at times feel that you wish to swear or hit someone because your anger is so great. This anger may be frightening to you, if it is something that you are not accustomed to feeling. You may not recognize or know how to handle these angry feelings. Many women also are angry at themselves for something that they did or did not do during the assault. These feelings of anger directed at yourself may lead to feelings of blame, guilt, helplessness, and depression. Many women also find that they are experiencing anger and irritability towards those people that they love the most: family, friends, their partners, and their children. It may be especially confusing for you to feel angry at those closest to you. This reaction may occur because anger needs an object for expression and may therefore attach itself to those people most available to us. Anger can also arise from a feeling that the world is not fair. This anger is not surprising in that the assault may have turned your assumptions about life upside down.

Has this been happening to you?

Sometimes you might *lose your temper* with the people who are most dear to you. This may be confusing because you may not understand why you are most angry and irritable with those you care about most. While closeness with others may feel good, it also increases the opportunity for feelings of intimacy, dependency, and vulnerability and helplessness. Having those feelings may make you feel angry and irritable because they remind you of the assault. We also may expect more from the people we love and get angry when they disappoint us. Sometimes, we just "let loose" with our family and friends our emotions and reactions that we hide from others.

10. After the assault, many individuals suffer a lowering of their *self-image.* You may tell yourself "I am a bad person and bad things happen to me," or "If I had not been so weak or stupid, this would not have happened to me," or "I should have been tougher." Many women see themselves as more negative overall after the assault and may tell themselves "I am a bad person and deserved this."

Are you having any negative thoughts about yourself since the assault? What kinds of things do you find yourself saying or thinking about your feelings or the way you are coping?

11. *Disruptions in relationships* with other people are not unusual after an assault. This disruption is in part due to feeling angry, scared, and depressed. You may isolate yourself from interacting with other people or not participate in the activities that you once did, in an effort to deal with the negative emotions you are experiencing. You may expect loved ones to offer the most help and support, yet find that they don't. It is also very common to see others more negatively, and to feel that you can't *trust* anyone. If you previously viewed the world as safe, the assault brings the realization that the world is dangerous. If you had previous bad experiences, the assault convinces you that the world is dangerous and

others aren't to be trusted. These negative thoughts often make women feel they have been changed completely by the assault. Relationships with others can become tense and it is difficult to become intimate with people as your trust decreases.

Have you had problems trusting other people? Do you have trouble getting along with others?

People frequently experience anger, anguish, and guilt when people that they love are hurt. Your friends and relatives, especially your partner, may have difficulty hearing about your assault and may have serious reactions to it. Although it is important that you get support for what you are going through, it is also important that you understand that some of the people around you might also be going through a crisis related to your assault. Imagine how you would feel if this happened to your daughter. You might be so upset that someone could do this to her, so blinded by rage, that you may not be as attentive to her needs. Sometimes we need to learn to forgive others' reactions to us when they don't give us what we need. In the long run, the support of your family and friends plays an important role in your recovery. A good strategy is to talk to people who you feel can support you and understand your feelings while being patient with those who may themselves need more time. If you have not found anyone who you can talk to about the assault, you may consult with your therapist about this situation or call a rape crisis center to learn of any support groups that exist in your area.

12. You may also have a *loss of interest in physical affection and sexual relations* following the assault. It is a common reaction for women to lose interest in sex if they are depressed, even though they might not have been assaulted. Also, disinterest in or fear of physical and sexual relations is extremely common in women who have been sexually assaulted. Intimacy and sexual relations may remind them of the assault.

Have you experienced any loss of interest in sexual relations? Do you have any frightening feelings, thoughts, or flashbacks during physical contact with anyone? Please write these in your notebook.

You may feel uncomfortable being emotionally and sexually intimate with someone because this experience may bring back your feelings of vulnerability during the assault. In fact, you may have flashbacks or intensely upsetting feelings when you are having sexual or physical contact.

13. You may find yourself remembering *past experiences*. Once a negative experience comes to your mind, it may trigger memories of other negative experiences. This happens because the way memories are stored may be related to the feeling they create. For this reason, you may find that following the trauma you may recall many negative memories about

a past trauma that you had forgotten. These memories may be as disturbing to you as the memories of your more recent assault.

The assault may be the reason you are recollecting bad experiences from your past and you may have problems in trying to bring to mind anything positive. In fact, it may be very difficult to believe that you will ever feel happy again or have pleasant experiences. But you will. In fact, you will begin to recall more positive experiences and put the negative memories behind you. The positive memories will trigger more positive recollections and eventually you will gain a more balanced view of your life.

Have you suddenly remembered upsetting experiences that you had before the assault? Please write these down.

Thoughts of Harming

Thoughts about harming oneself or an assailant are relatively common among rape survivors. If you are experiencing any of these thoughts, they are very significant and need to be addressed in therapy.

Do you have any thoughts, urges, feelings, fantasies, and plans to harm yourself? Have you ever thought about or planned to hurt yourself in the past? How serious was the attempt? Do you have any intention of carrying out these plans now or in the near future? Do you have lethal means available to you? For example, do you have enough pills or a gun?

If you are actively considering suicide, or if you answered "yes" to any of the questions above about suicide, we urge you to talk to your therapist about this. This is too serious to try and handle it on your own. If you have these thoughts after you have finished therapy, you should call your therapist and make an appointment. If you cannot afford to see someone privately or this service is not covered in your insurance or you do not have insurance, you can call your local Mental Health Association and find out where an agency is near you and how to make an appointment.

Although it will be difficult, please tell the intake person that you are having suicidal thoughts, because they will need to know that to get you in as quickly as possible. If you have not been able to make an appointment and you are actively considering suicide, please call 911 and tell them and they will help.

As therapists, we have found that all our clients who considered suicide were glad at a later date that they did not kill themselves. Most suicidal people do not really want to be dead, they just want to stop the pain they feel and cannot come up with constructive solutions. We know it is easy for others to stand back and say you have a reason to live, because they are not feeling your pain and despair. But we do know from working with so many survivors that these feelings can pass and you can feel better again, but it will take some work on your part. Many people look back on these periods in their life and wonder how they made it through them, but they are glad they did.

Many survivors have expressed thoughts of harming their assailants as well. Statements such as "If they find him, I'll kill him" or "I want to make him suffer like he made me suffer" are common reactions to assault. We have never actually had an assault survivor who then harmed her assailant, but it does happen, especially in partner abuse.

Do you have access to your assailant? Do you really *plan* to harm him, not just think about it? How would you do it, if you really intended to harm him? Do you have access to weapons or other means of harming him?

If you answered "yes" to any of these questions about intending to harm your assailant, again, we urge you to discuss this with your therapist. If this occurs after you have completed therapy, call your therapist back for an appointment. We urge you to see a professional and to tell her or him openly about your ideas and plans. These thoughts are too serious also to deal with on your own. Although such thoughts may not be uncommon among survivors, acting on them is not a solution and can only make matters much worse for you.

Some of the common reactions to an assault are connected with each other. For some people, having a flashback may increase their concern about losing control of their lives and may even make their fears worse. In other words, the responses of being assaulted often interact with one another and cause the overall response to be more intense. Of all the normal reactions to assault, fear is probably the most common and appears to be the most debilitating. It is important to know that as you become aware of the changes you have gone through since the assault, and as you process these experiences during treatment, the symptoms should become less upsetting.

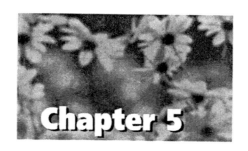

Chapter 5

Assessing My PTSD

Assessment of My Problems

In the previous chapter, we presented many of the common reactions to assault. If you are following the program as you read this workbook, you may have written down some of the problems you have been experiencing. In this chapter, you may take the next step in the program and think about the various symptoms of PTSD you may be experiencing. Identifying these symptoms will help you and your therapist decide which of them to observe or monitor throughout your program as an indication of whether the program is helping you to work through your PTSD.

The first step in assessing whether you are suffering from PTSD is to determine if you have been a survivor of a trauma. Have you been in any situation in which you felt you were likely to be killed or seriously injured? The following is a list of examples of traumatic events. If you have experienced more than one trauma, please rank order them in terms of how much each is disturbing you at the present time. Mark the most disturbing trauma with a "1." Mark the next most disturbing trauma with a "2" and so on.

Examples of Traumas

If you have experienced a type of trauma more than once (e.g., having had two car accidents), rank it only once for how much it disturbed you:

___ A *serious* accident at work, in a car, or somewhere else

___ A natural disaster such as a tornado, hurricane, flood, major earthquake

___ Seeing someone seriously injured or violently killed

___ Being seriously injured yourself

___ A situation in which you feared you might be seriously injured or killed

___ Accidental death of a family member as a result of a crime

___ Other accidental death of a family member

___ Forced sex (putting a penis in your vagina)

___ Forced other sexual contact (putting penis, tongue, or other objects in vagina, anus, or mouth)

___ Forced/unwanted sexual touching/fondling

___ Physical attack with a weapon

___ Physical attack without a weapon

___ Physical assault (beat up)

___ Survivor of a crime

___ Kidnapped

___ Other (please list:_____)

If you have checked any of the events, you have experienced a traumatic event. Any and all events checked above should be discussed with your therapist. The severity of disturbance associated with the event(s) can be further assessed in discussion with your therapist.

Rating of Posttraumatic Stress Disorder Symptoms

The second step in assessing PTSD is identifying symptoms. Below is a description of the PTSD symptoms. Please rate each symptom that you are currently experiencing on a 0–3 scale. "0" indicates that you do not have this symptom or that it is so mild that it is not at all a problem for you; "1" indicates it is a mild problem for you; "2" indicates it is a moderate problem for you; and "3" indicates it is a severe problem for you. It would be helpful to complete this now, and again at the end of treatment, so please write down your responses below:

0 = not a problem

1 = mild problem

2 = moderate problem

3 = severe problem

I. Reexperiencing the traumatic event:

___ 1. Thoughts, images, or ideas about the trauma that keep coming back and are unwanted and cause distress

___ 2. Nightmares or bad dreams about the trauma or that seem related to it

___ 3. Flashbacks of the traumatic event, as if it were happening again

___ 4. Extreme emotional distress when I am reminded of the traumatic event

___ 5. Extreme bodily reactions when I am reminded of the traumatic event (for example, heart races, get sweaty, tense up)

II. Continual avoidance of reminders of the traumatic event and/or emotional numbing:

___ 1. Avoid thinking about, talking about, or feelings associated with the trauma

___ 2. Avoid situations, activities, places, or people that remind me of the traumatic event

___ 3. Can't remember *important* parts of what happened

___ 4. Large decrease in interest or time spent in activities that were important to me

___ 5. Feeling cut off from or like I can't connect with other people

___ 6. Emotional numbing; don't experience the whole range of emotions that I used to

___ 7. Feel my life will be cut short; don't expect to live as long as I had thought

III. Indications of increased arousal:

___ 1. Continual problems falling or staying asleep

___ 2. Extreme irritability or outbursts of anger

___ 3. Persistent difficulty concentrating

___ 4. Extreme "scanning" of environment, checking the situation all around me, hypervigilant

___ 5. Extremely jumpy, startle very easily

Note. Reprinted with permission from the *Diagnostic and Statistical Manual of Mental Disorders, Fourth Edition.* Copyright 1994 American Psychiatric Association.

Please discuss your experience of these symptoms with your therapist. If you do not experience any or many of these problems, you may not need to have treatment for PTSD. However, if a number of these symptoms are a problem for you, and/or you experience any of them to a severe degree, this treatment program is likely to help you. Once you and your therapist have decided to start treatment, you need to continue with careful assessment. This is discussed below.

Usefulness of Assessment

The assessment above can help you and your therapist determine the need for treatment. In addition, assessment is an important part of the preparation for treatment, as ongoing monitoring during treatment, and as a method to determine your response to treatment. Often, survivors do not connect many of their current problems to the assault even when in fact they do result from the assault. Instead, they may feel as if they are going crazy or losing the ability to cope. If you are able to start linking many problems to the assault, it may help you to become more aware and start to feel that at least your reactions are expected and common to this type of experience. Think back to when you've been sick: if you were informed that the side effects of the medication that you took included stomach upset, then you were probably much less worried when you experienced stomach upset than if you thought that there was yet another thing wrong with you. It helps to know what to expect and what it's caused by. For example, it may help to notice some regular patterns or triggers to your problems, making your reactions more predictable and your feelings seem less crazy.

Assessment is also important in helping you and your therapist understand how severe your problems are. Progress in treatment can be measured against this baseline, or level of symptom severity that you experienced before treatment. Even if you are not as far along as you would like after going through this program, it may be useful to compare where you are with where you used to be. Many individuals find it encouraging to realize that more progress has been made than they are aware of. For example, if a survivor is disheartened because she still feels jumpy occasionally, it will help to realize that before treatment this was happening daily, whereas now it occurs less than weekly.

There are many methods of assessment, all of which have advantages and disadvantages. Self-monitoring involves your recording each time the troublesome symptom (e.g., nightmares) occurs. The most common form involves indicating on a sheet of paper the number of occurrences of the identified symptom as well as other relevant information, including the date and time, situation, thoughts, and reactions (Figure 5.1 is a self-monitoring form. A sample of a completed form is shown in Figure 5.2). Reactions may be recorded as SUDS, or Subjective Units of Discomfort, rated on a 0–100 scale in which "0" indicates no anxiety or discomfort and "100" indicates panic level anxiety or discomfort.

It is important to record the date and time in order to determine patterns of problems. This process may reveal specific times when you may be at higher risk for strong reactions. For many rape survivors nighttime is more difficult. The situation (e.g., location, others present, activity) is also important in figuring out common triggers. A survivor may say that it scares her to go to the grocery store, but it may be that it scares her when she goes to a certain store at night by herself, but she's not bothered by other stores or at other times of the day or when accompanied.

Self-monitoring is important for judging your response to treatment and increasing your awareness of the problems and their patterns. Other methods of self-monitoring include counting the number of occurrences of the symptoms, for example using a pocket counter or tic marks, duration ratings (i.e., how long strong reactions last), or asking someone close to you to rate your reactions.

Self-Monitoring Form

Target Behaviors

Target Behavior A: _____

Target Behavior B: _____

Date & Time	Situation	Thoughts	Target Behavior	SUDS

Figure 5.1.

Self-Monitoring Form

Target Behaviors

Target Behavior A: *nightmares*

Target Behavior B: *angry outbursts*

Target Behaviors

Date & Time	Situation	Thoughts	Target Behavior	SUDS
7/7 2 AM	in bed	I'm scared	A	80
7/7 7:30 AM	getting kids ready	They're driving me crazy	B	75
7/9 3:30 AM	in bed	not again	A	60
7/10 8:00 PM	kids in bath	they're too slow	B	50

Figure 5.2.   **Example of Self-Monitoring**

Advantages of self-monitoring include getting an accurate account of the symptoms and related information, increasing your awareness of symptoms and problematic situations, and teaching yourself to think in contextual terms (that is, the context in which a certain behavior occurs). As an ongoing measure throughout treatment, self-monitoring is valuable. If you find it inconvenient to carry your self-monitoring sheet with you, you can note any occurrence of the target behavior on any available paper and then transfer it to the self-monitoring sheet when you get home. Be creative! Refer back to the notes you made on yourself from the previous chapter to help decide, with your therapist, what would be good targets for self-monitoring. Some suggestions for target behaviors for self-monitoring are found on Table 5.1:

Table 5.1.   **Examples of Target Behaviors**

Intrusive thoughts of the assault

Flashbacks of the assault

Nightmares related to the assault

Instances of strong emotional reactions to reminders of the assault

Instances of strong physical reactions to reminders of the assault

Exaggerated startle reactions

Instances of excessive irritability or anger

Sleep disturbances

Hypervigilant responses

Problems concentrating

The avoidance/numbing symptoms, including avoiding reminders of the assault, feeling cut off from others, decreased interest in activities, sense of a shortened future, and not remembering the entire experience, are more difficult to self-monitor because they often do not occur in distinct episodes and often are not as easy to recognize.

It is sometimes difficult to determine which symptoms to monitor. Nightmares? Avoidance? Flashbacks? Depression? You and your therapist must determine the particular symptoms to monitor. What are the most troubling symptoms for you? What's happening the most frequently? What are the first problems you think of when you think of the problems you're currently having as a result of the assault? Remember, symptoms can be behaviors, such as avoiding feared places. If, after careful self-monitoring, it appears you chose incorrectly, you can change the target symptoms or behaviors for monitoring. However, remember that the true evidence of progress in treatment of a specific symptom requires a baseline or beginning measure of that symptom at the start of treatment. Do not make the mistake of switching symptoms "with the wind" if you are experiencing different symptoms each week. Keep in mind the fact that when the main symptoms are not as problematic, previously minor symptoms may seem worse because the more serious symptoms are gone. Although it is not useful to switch the symptoms for self-monitoring to these previously minor symptoms, you can add them to the list so you can monitor your progress with those, as well, if you wish.

Other Problems Associated with Assault

Depression

It is common to feel sad and depressed following an assault, but is your depression severe enough that it requires treatment of its own? Please assess yourself with the following checklist:

For most of the day, almost every day, have you experienced any of the following symptoms: (check all that apply)

___ 1. Your mood is blue or depressed

___ 2. You have trouble concentrating or making a decision

___ 3. You have frequent thoughts of death, suicide, or a suicide attempt

___ 4. You have feelings of worthlessness or excessive guilt

___ 5. You have sleep problems (either insomnia or sleeping too much)

___ 6. You have lost weight when not trying to diet

___ 7. You do not have interest or find pleasure in daily activities

___ 8. You are physically restless or physically slowed down

___ 9. Your energy is low almost every day

If you checked 5 or more of the above symptoms, you may be suffering from a *major depressive episode.* Please discuss this with your therapist. There are good treatments for depression that can help you feel better. If you answered a few questions positively but not enough to indicate a major depressive episode, you may still profit from treatment for depression. However, it is very common for assault survivors with PTSD to also feel a little depressed. Usually, when the PTSD improves, the depression does also. If, after completing the program described in this book, your depression has not improved, please discuss this with your therapist.

Substance Abuse or Dependence

Do you have a problem with drugs or alcohol? Even prescription medications? Please assess yourself with the following checklist:

Have you experienced any of the following symptoms: (check all that apply)

___ 1. You need increasingly more of the substance to achieve the same effect

___ 2. You experience unpleasant symptoms when not using the substance (for example, shakes in the morning)

___ 3. You use more of the substance than you intended

___ 4. Your efforts to stop or cut down use in the past have not worked

___ 5. You are spending a lot of your time and energy getting the drugs or alcohol, or a lot of time taking it, or a lot of time recovering from it, or all three

___ 6. Your substance use has led you to give up important activities in your life

___ 7. You continue to use the drug or alcohol even when you know it is causing you harm

If you checked 3 or more of the above symptoms, you may be suffering from a *substance dependence disorder*. Please discuss this with your therapist.

Have you experienced any of the following symptoms: (check all that apply)

___ 1. You continue to use alcohol or drugs even though they have interfered with your responsibilities (for example, absences or tardiness or poor performance at work, school, or home)

___ 2. You continue to use in situations in which it is dangerous (for example, driving a car while intoxicated)

___ 3. You have had legal problems related to the substance use (for example, driving under the influence)

___ 4. Your relationships have suffered (for example, arguments with spouse, fights) and still you continue to use

If you checked any of the above symptoms, you may be suffering from a *substance abuse disorder*. Please discuss this with your therapist. Many trauma survivors use alcohol and drugs as a means of avoidance. Most professionals think that you have to quit using drugs or drinking alcohol to adequately process the trauma. If you have a substance abuse or dependence disorder, you may have difficulty stopping on your own. We urge you to discuss this with your therapist. If you answered a few questions positively but not enough to indicate a substance abuse or dependence disorder, you may still profit from drug and alcohol treatment. We urge you to discontinue use of alcohol and drugs while you are using the procedures described in this book to be able to fully gain from them. At the least, you should drastically reduce the use of alcohol and drugs. If you are not able to reduce or stop, that would be an indication you need additional help.

Other Problems

In Chapter 3 we described a number of other problems that can result from an assault, including sexual problems, relationship problems, and dissociative reactions. If you feel that any of these are causing you significant distress and are interfering in your life, you may require additional treatment for that problem. If you are unsure, please discuss these problems with your therapist. Most problems can be handled one step at a time. Your therapist can help you understand which steps you should take first.

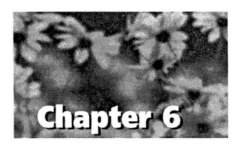

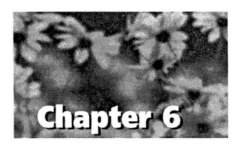Chapter 6

What Do We Know About the Treatment of PTSD?

In this chapter, we will summarize the knowledge that comes from studies on the treatment of PTSD, psychological therapy and therapy by medication. We will begin with a brief review of traditional therapies for PTSD. This review is by no means comprehensive and is intended as an introduction. If you want to find out more about these approaches, you can look up the references pertaining to a topic in the Additional Reading section of this chapter. We will also briefly review a few of the large number of studies on cognitive-behavioral treatment programs for PTSD, which is the treatment program described in this workbook. We have included some discussions of treatment with survivors of traumas other than sexual assault as there are many similarities in the problems and treatment of PTSD across traumas. In our review here we will discuss results of studies comparing the effectiveness of different treatment programs, and we will also discuss case reports that clearly describe the treatment and evaluate the efficacy of the treatment with good measures. Results of studies in which some clients are given treatment soon after they present to the clinic are compared with others who receive a delayed treatment after first being put on a wait-list. The effectiveness of treatment is often determined by comparing clients who received the treatment to those on the wait-list.

In our opinion, it is important that you know how to judge the effectiveness of a treatment program that you undertake. Unfortunately, not all studies of PTSD treatments are well-controlled, meaning that we can't be sure how to interpret the results. The more well-controlled a study is, the stronger are the conclusions that can be drawn from its results. In contrast, the results of less-controlled studies are open to various explanations and are therefore less conclusive.

Crisis Intervention and Acute Posttraumatic Stress

Crisis intervention and supportive group therapy centered on trauma survivors are the approaches used in rape crisis centers. Crisis counseling focuses on providing information, active listening, and emotional support. Although frequently used, no well-controlled studies have been conducted on these techniques to establish their effectiveness.

Even though no research has been conducted on rape crisis centers, they do provide very valuable services. Many rape crisis centers provide immediate assistance, often being called in by the police or emergency room when a rape is reported. Many provide a hot line for 24-hour availability. This rapid availability can be very helpful for a person who may be in a state of shock immediately following an assault.

Rape crisis center counselors are there to assist the survivor with information, protection, support, and crisis counseling, which also opens the door for possible future intervention. The support groups provide a forum for survivors to feel accepted and heard and to recognize they are not alone. It is often easier for survivors to recognize that someone else who was assaulted did nothing wrong than to see this for themselves. Support groups in rape crisis centers may help provide survivors this perspective. In addition, many, if not most, rape crisis centers provide their services free of charge and thus are an invaluable resource. Rape crisis centers have provided services to multitudes of women over the years. Their counselors and directors are some of our communities' unsung heroes.

Although many survivors who receive crisis intervention report help with pain of the immediate reaction, the longer term development of PTSD may not be prevented. The following study found that the cognitive-behavioral treatment program discussed in this workbook was effective in preventing prolonged PTSD symptoms.

Foa and her colleagues in 1995 conducted a study of a brief prevention program (BP) for female assault survivors. Included in this treatment were imaginal exposure, relaxation training, and cognitive restructuring (these techniques will be described in detail in later chapters of this book). This program helped the majority of the women in it substantially and seemed to prevent the development of PTSD in many.

In summary, although there is no research on crisis interventions, rape crisis centers clearly provide important services. With female assault survivors, short-term behavioral interventions may help in preventing chronic posttrauma problems.

Traditional Therapies

Hypnotherapy

The use of hypnosis in the treatment of trauma-related problems goes back at least to Freud (for a review, see Spiegel, 1989) who introduced the procedure to produce the psychological release of emotion he thought was necessary to resolve a psychic conflict. The theory is that hypnosis may allow recall of traumatic events that are not available to conscious recollection. A number of case reports have described the usefulness of hypnosis in treating PTSD. One controlled study that examined the efficacy of hypnosis was conducted by Brom, Kleber, and Defres in 1989. The result of this study suggests that hypnotherapy offered some help for posttrauma suffering.

Psychodynamic Treatments

Psychodynamic theories emphasize concepts of defense, emotional release and expression, as well as stages of recovery from trauma in developing treatment for posttrauma difficulties. The target of Horowitz's brief psychodynamic therapy (Horowitz, 1976) is the resolution of intra-psychic conflict arising from a traumatic experience. Some studies, one headed by Lindy in 1983 and another by Roth in 1988, show that psychodynamic treatments may be useful in the treatment of PTSD. See the Additional Reading section for further information. However, none of these studies are well-controlled and thus our knowledge of how well this type of treatment works is limited.

Cognitive-Behavioral Therapy

The most frequently studied psychological treatments for PTSD are the cognitive-behavioral programs. These treatments include a number of different techniques and programs, including exposure programs, cognitive restructuring, anxiety management programs, and their combinations. You will understand more about what these terms mean as you read through the rest of the workbook. Cognitive-behavioral treatments typically have been tested by assessing the target symptoms such as PTSD before and after therapy, by having comparison groups, and by using well-described procedures. These techniques will be described in detail in later chapters, whereas this chapter will present an overview of the studies.

Exposure

One type of cognitive-behavioral program that has been used for PTSD sufferers is exposure therapy. Exposure therapy helps clients to confront situations, objects, and memories that cause them to be very anxious and distressed and interfere with their daily functioning. When exposure is conducted in imagination, we call it imaginal exposure; when it is conducted in real life, we call it in vivo exposure. For PTSD, imaginal exposure usually involves having the person relive the trauma in her imagination and describe it out loud, over and over and over again, until it becomes less painful. The use of imaginal exposure techniques requires that the person remember at least some details of the trauma and is aware of some of the triggers for the traumatic memory. Programs that focus on exposure have the most evidence for their effectiveness.

Both exposure in imagination and exposure in real life to trauma reminders are very helpful in reducing PTSD and related problems. An example of exposure treatment that we have developed over the years asks the client to recall the traumatic memories in the therapist's office. The client is asked to go back in her mind to the time of the trauma and to relive it in her imagination. She is asked to close her eyes and to describe it out loud in the present tense, as if it were happening now. Typically, the story is tape-recorded (audiotaped) and that tape is sent home with the client so that she may practice imaginal exposure by listening to the tape at home, preferably daily, between therapy sessions. Although this reliving can be distressing initially, it quickly becomes less painful as exposure is repeated. The idea behind this type of treatment is that the trauma needs to be emotionally processed, or digested, so that it can become less painful. The process is similar to the grief process: losing a loved one causes extreme pain for the survivors, but by expressing that pain (say through crying and talking about the deceased), the pain gradually subsides. Eventually, we can think about that person without crying, although the loss will always be sad.

Another form of exposure involves actually confronting repeatedly, in real-life safe situations, places, or objects that are reminders of the trauma until they no longer evoke anxiety. Some therapists use exposure in the form of having the client write repeatedly about the trauma. In systematic desensitization, the person is taught how to relax, then presented with reminders of the trauma gradually, working up a hierarchy from the least disturbing reminder to the most disturbing reminder. If the individual becomes too anxious or upset, she may relax, then go back to the image for exposure. This process is repeated until she can confront all memories or situations without becoming upset.

Several forms of exposure treatment have been developed for anxiety disorders, all involving the common feature of having participants confront their fears. The effectiveness of exposure treatment for PTSD was first demonstrated with several case reports on war veterans. Both exposure in imagination and exposure in vivo to trauma related events appeared to be helpful.

Systematic Desensitization

Some of the earliest studies of behavioral treatments for PTSD used the systematic desensitization (SD) technique pioneered by Wolpe (1958). SD was moderately helpful in two studies with war veterans, but a large number of sessions over a long period of time were required. Several uncontrolled studies demonstrated that SD was effective with rape survivors in reducing fear, anxiety, depression, and social maladjustment. Thus, most studies showed that SD can be somewhat helpful for survivors of different traumas. However, most of the studies were not well-controlled and/or did not include PTSD diagnoses and measures, so the conclusions that we can draw from these studies are limited.

Prolonged Imaginal and In Vivo Exposure

For the most part, SD is not used anymore as a treatment for anxiety disorders, including PTSD. As noted earlier, current exposure programs for PTSD involve repeated reliving of the trauma, and trying to help process the trauma. We think that exposure helps PTSD by allowing participants to realize that: (a) just because they are reminded of the assault, it does not mean they are in danger; (b) remembering the assault is not the same as having it happen again; (c) anxiety will eventually come down, even when they stay with the feared situations or memories; and (d) experiencing anxiety/PTSD symptoms does not lead to loss of control. It is through these steps that traumatic events may be emotionally processed, and emotionally digested. By bringing up the traumatic memory and going over and over it, this allows the memory to be processed, which allows the survivor to move on. For more information on this, see *Treating the Trauma of Rape: Cognitive-Behavioral Therapy for PTSD* by Foa and Rothbaum.

In a 1991 study with sexual assault survivors who suffered chronic PTSD, Foa and Rothbaum and their colleagues compared prolonged exposure with other types of therapy. They randomly assigned participants to one of three treatment conditions: prolonged exposure (PE, including both imaginal and in vivo exposure), stress inoculation training (SIT), or supportive counseling (SC). To assess progress using these treatments, those treated were compared to those in a wait-list control condition. Immediately following treatment, both SIT and PE participants improved on all clusters of PTSD symptoms (i.e., reexperiencing, avoidance, and arousal). Participants receiving supportive counseling or on the wait-list improved on the arousal symptoms of PTSD, but not on the avoidance or reexperiencing symptoms. At follow-up, PE appeared the most successful. A second study by Foa and colleagues compared PE, SIT, and the combination of SIT and PE, to a wait-list control. In this study, all three active treatments were quite helpful in reducing PTSD and depression; clients in the wait-list did not improve. On some measures, but not on others, PE produced results superior to the other treatments. Three other studies also found imaginal and in vivo exposure treatment helpful for PTSD for participants having experienced various traumas. Complete listings for these studies can be found in the Additional Reading section.

The results from many studies consistently support the effectiveness of imaginal and in vivo exposure for the treatment of PTSD. Many of these studies were well-controlled, and therefore we can have confidence in the results. If you'd like to know more about these studies, see *Treating the Trauma of Rape: Cognitive-Behavioral Therapy for PTSD* (Rothbaum & Foa, 1998).

Eye Movement Desensitization and Reprocessing

A new technique, Eye Movement Desensitization and Reprocessing (EMDR) is a form of exposure (desensitization) accompanied by eye movements. Briefly, the technique involves the client's imagining a scene from the trauma, focusing on the thoughts and feelings that go with that picture, while the client follows the therapist's fingers moving back and forth in front of her eyes (Shapiro, 1995). This is repeated until anxiety decreases, at which point the client is instructed to generate a more adaptive thought and to associate it with the scene while moving her eyes.

EMDR has been controversial for a number of reasons, including claims by its originator that it worked in a single session. A number of case studies have reported positive findings. Several studies have found EMDR to be successful; some have had mixed results, and some have not shown EMDR to be more successful than control treatments. In general, the studies of EMDR indicate reduction in anxiety during the therapy session, but the clear efficacy of this treatment with PTSD has been demonstrated only in the Rothbaum (1997) study. Some studies found improvement with EMDR but were not well-controlled. Other results question the role of the eye movements. One recent study conducted by Devilly and Spence compared EMDR with a program that included PE and some components of SIT. The results showed that PE/SIT was superior to EMDR, especially at a three-month follow-up: clients that received SIT/PE retained their improvement but clients that received EMDR tended to relapse.

Anxiety Management Programs

Anxiety management training (AMT) programs include relaxation training, positive self-statements, breathing retraining, biofeedback, social skills training, and distraction techniques. The goal of AMT is to give clients ways to manage anxiety when it occurs. Anxiety management training has also been helpful with PTSD. Here, the focus is on the management of fear, generally by teaching clients skills to control their anxiety. One of the most common anxiety management programs for PTSD is stress inoculation training (SIT; see the Kilpatrick and Veronen study in 1983 for more information). SIT typically consists of education and training of coping skills. These skills include muscle relaxation training, breathing control, role-playing, covert modeling, thought-stopping, and guided self-dialogue (Meichenbaum, 1975). The idea is that sufferers of PTSD experience a great deal of anxiety and stress in their lives. Very often, when clients become anxious, they take it as a sign that they are facing danger and, thus, they become even more scared.

The benefits of SIT for female rape survivors have been supported by several studies. The results indicated that SIT was effective in reducing rape-related fear, anxiety, and avoidance, as well as general tension and depression and most of these gains were maintained after treatment ended. As described above, our studies found SIT to be effective, but on some measures it was less effective than exposure.

In summary, the effectiveness of SIT for reducing PTSD and related symptoms was supported by controlled studies. However, all of these studies were conducted with female assault survivors, and thus the effectiveness of SIT for other trauma populations is still unknown.

Combined Treatment Programs

Because both Stress Inoculation Training and Prolonged Exposure seemed so helpful, experts believed that combining these programs would help even more. Specifically, it was thought that a combined program will help trauma survivors confront what they are scared of, while also giving them ways to manage stress and anxiety. The effectiveness of two such programs have been studied for PTSD in women with assault-related PTSD. The first of these studies by Foa and her colleagues has already been discussed. Briefly, the combined treatment did not seem to help any more than each of the treatments alone, and was, perhaps, not even as good as exposure alone. Because the combined treatment was delivered in the same number and length of sessions, clients who received this treatment did not get as much imaginal exposure as the PE group, nor did they receive as much SIT as in the SIT group. This might explain the failure of the combined program to show more benefit than the single-component treatments; in many ways, they got less of each treatment. However, a modification of this program was very effective in reducing PTSD symptoms in a study with motor vehicle accident survivors.

Another combined treatment approach, Cognitive Processing Therapy (CPT; for more information, see the Resick and Schnicke 1992 study), was designed specifically for rape survivors and has been shown to help PTSD and depression. Exposure therapy in CPT is accomplished through writing about the rape and then reading the account in a group therapy situation. Cognitive therapy in CPT focuses on five themes: safety, trust, power, esteem, and intimacy. CPT was found quite effective in reducing PTSD symptoms compared to a wait-list condition, but the study was not controlled. In an ongoing controlled study, Resick and her colleagues are comparing PE and CPT. Preliminary results suggest that both programs are highly effective and do not differ from one another.

In summary, so far it does not appear that combination treatments are better than PE or SIT alone. However, it may be this is due to the combination actually reducing the time for SIT and PE, as discussed earlier.

Pharmacological Treatments

Studies of medications for PTSD suggest that antidepressant drugs of three different classes have therapeutic effects that are significantly greater than nonspecific effects of a placebo. Most have helped at least somewhat, although sometimes not more so than placebo. Tricyclic antidepressants and selective serotonin reuptake inhibitors (SSRIs) seem to be effective for PTSD, but the effects of other drugs are less clear. The benefits of the SSRIs have been the most impressive.

The Selective Serotonin Reuptake Inhibitors (SSRI) include Prozac® (fluoxetine), Zoloft® (sertraline), Paxil® (paroxetine), and Luvox® (fluvoxamine). Two large, well-controlled studies have found sertraline effective and safe for survivors with PTSD from various traumas. Open studies and one controlled study have suggested fluoxetine to be effective in PTSD, both among combat veterans and sexual assault survivors. There are no controlled studies examining the effects of medication for PTSD in female rape survivors, but an open trial found sertraline effective for 80% of rape survivors studied. At this point in time, SSRIs seem to be the choice medication group among antidepressants and the most promising for PTSD. A medication similar to an SSRI called Serzone® (nefazodone) has been shown in preliminary reports to be helpful for PTSD.

In general, medications should be considered only when the PTSD symptoms have persisted for several weeks and seem to have become chronic. It seems that a minimum of 5 to 8 weeks of taking antidepressant medication is required to begin to get full effects. And, it may be that several months of an antidepressant may lead to more improvement. Reports from the 1996 study conducted by Rothbaum and colleagues using sertraline with PTSD rape survivors, indicate that some of the participants were able to deal better with the assault once on medication and were able to discontinue the medication successfully. They reported being able to talk about the assault more and work on it in ongoing therapy. It may be that the medication decreased their PTSD symptoms, and allowed them to work on processing the trauma. Once the trauma was adequately processed, these individuals no longer required the medication.

In this chapter we have discussed the effectiveness of techniques in treating PTSD and related problems in different trauma populations. Different types of treatments have appeared to be helpful, although the number of studies showing the effectiveness of cognitive-behavior therapy is greater than the number of studies showing the efficacy of other approaches.

Additional Reading

Brom, D., Kleber, R. J., & Defares, P. B. (1989). Brief psychotherapy for posttraumatic stress disorders. *Journal of Consulting and Clinical Psychology, 57*(5), 607-612.

Devilly, G. J. & Spence, S. H. (in press). The relative efficacy and treatment distress of EMDR and a cognitive behavioral trauma treatment protocol in the amelioration of post-traumatic stress disorder. *Journal of Anxiety Disorders.*

Foa, E. B., Dancu, C. V., Hembree, E., Jaycox, L. H., Meadows, E. A., & Street, G. P. (1999). The efficacy of exposure therapy, stress inoculation training and their combination in ameliorating PTSD for female survivors of assault. *Journal of Consulting and Clinical Psychology, 67*(2), 194-200.

Foa, E. B., Hearst-Ikeda, D. E., & Perry, K. J. (1995). Evaluation of a brief cognitive-behavioral program for the prevention of chronic PTSD in recent assault survivors. *Journal of Consulting and Clinical Psychology 63*(6), 948-955.

Foa, E. B. & Rothbaum, B. O. (1998). *Treating the trauma of rape: Cognitive-behavioral therapy for PTSD.* New York: Guilford Press.

Foa, E. B., Rothbaum, B.O., Riggs, D. S., & Murdock, T.B. (1991). Treatment of posttraumatic stress disorder in rape survivors: A comparison between cognitive-behavioral procedures and counseling. *Journal of Consulting and Clinical Psychology, 59*(5), 715-723.

Horowitz, M. J. (1976). *Stress response syndromes.* New York: Jason Aronson Inc.

Kilpatrick, D. G., & Veronen, L. J. (1983). Treatment for rape-related problems: Crisis intervention is not enough. In L. Cohen, W. Claiborn & G. Specter (Eds.), *Crisis Intervention* (2nd ed.). New York: Human Sciences Press.

Lindy, J. D., Green, B. L., Grace, M., & Titchener, J. (1983). Psychotherapy with survivors of the Beverly Hills Supper Club fire. *American Journal of Psychotherapy, 37*(4), 593-610.

Marks, I., Lovell, K., Noshirvani, H., Livanou, M., & Thrasher, S. (1998). Treatment of posttraumatic stress disorder by exposure and/or cognitive restructuring: A controlled study. *Archives of General Psychiatry, 55*(4), 317-325.

Meichenbaum, D. (1975). Self-instructional methods. In F. H. Kanfer & A. P. Goldstein (Eds.), *Helping people change: A textbook of methods.* New York: Pergamon Press.

Resick, P. A., & Schnicke, M. K. (1992). Cognitive processing therapy for sexual assault survivors. *Journal of Consulting and Clinical Psychology, 60*(5), 748-756.

Richards, D. A., Lovell, K., & Marks, I. M. (1994). Post-traumatic stress disorder: Evaluation of a behavioral treatment program. *Journal of Traumatic Stress, 7*(4), 669-680.

Roth, S., Dye, E., & Lebowitz, L. (1988). Group therapy for sexual-assault survivors. *Psychotherapy, 25*, 82-93.

Rothbaum, B. O. (1997). A controlled study of eye movement desensitization and reprocessing in the treatment of posttraumatic stress disordered sexual assault survivors. *Bulletin of the Menninger Clinic, 61*(3), 317-334.

Rothbaum, B. O., Ninan, P. T., & Thomas, L. (1996). Sertraline in the treatment of rape survivors with posttraumatic stress disorder. *Journal of Traumatic Stress, 9*(4), 865-871.

Shapiro, F. (1995). *Eye movement desensitization and reprocessing: Basic principles, protocols, and procedures.* New York: Guilford Press.

Spiegel, D. (1989). Hypnosis in the treatment of survivors of sexual abuse. *Psychiatric Clinics of North America, 12*(2), 295-305.

Thompson, J. A., Charlton, P. F., Kerry, R., Lee, D., & Turner, S. W. (1995). An open trial of exposure therapy based on deconditioning for post-traumatic stress disorder. *British Journal of Clinical Psychology, 34*(3), 407-416.

Wolpe, J. (1958). *Psychotherapy by reciprocal inhibition.* Stanford: Stanford University Press.

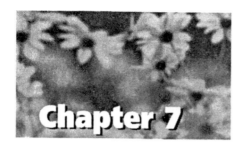

Chapter 7

Designing My Treatment Program

In this chapter, we will prepare for your treatment program. First, we will describe three program options. This sequence does not necessarily represent their relative benefit for you as a unique individual. You and your therapist will decide which is the best program for you. The specific treatment techniques are described in great detail in Sections IV and V. In these sections, the techniques are presented with Relaxation Training first. If you are not currently in therapy, this might be a good place to start.

Overview of Three Treatment Programs

In Section IV we will describe the cognitive-behavioral techniques that help with PTSD. These include exposure techniques and anxiety management procedures. We have found in our research that *prolonged exposure* (PE) alone (including trauma reliving and in vivo confrontation of trauma reminders) is as effective, if not more effective than more complicated programs. Therefore, we recommend the PE alone program as the first line of treatment for most survivors. We present the exposure program in a session-by-session format, because we recommend that everyone receive exposure therapy. We present each of the other techniques or set of techniques separately to teach all the cognitive-behavioral techniques that have been used with female assault survivors. You may not need all of the techniques that we describe here. Nevertheless three optional programs are outlined in this chapter.

Although PE alone may be the first line of treatment for many readers, we will first discuss exposure and *stress inoculation training* (SIT) for those readers for whom this is a more appropriate starting place.

1. Exposure and Stress Inoculation Training Program

For some survivors, a combination of exposure and SIT procedures is recommended. If you are very aroused (nervous, jittery) and feel out of control and/or extremely reluctant to expose yourself, it is possible to work on reducing this nervousness and increasing your sense of control through the stress inoculation techniques. The exposure techniques can be added at a later date, or begun when you feel ready for it. There are two main methods used in this treatment program. The first, exposure, both imaginal and in vivo, is the same as discussed in program 2. The second main strategy you will learn in this treatment program is called *anxiety management training*. This is a set of several techniques to help you control your anxiety. These include ways to relax your body, ways your thoughts can help you (cognitive techniques) and role-playing. After an assault, many survivors believe that the world is unpredictable and uncontrollable. They see the world as very dangerous. Thinking like this makes it hard to live a normal life. When you learn to identify these thoughts and change them, your symptoms should decrease. In summary, these techniques will give you skills to manage your anxiety and help you come to grips with what has happened to you.

2. Exposure Program

Many survivors, especially those with PTSD that involves mainly anxiety and avoidance symptoms, may be helped by the exposure program alone and would not need other programs.

The two main procedures of this treatment program are prolonged imaginal exposure and in vivo exposure. *Prolonged imaginal exposure* is intended to help you process the traumatic memory by asking you to relive the memory in your imagination repeatedly during the sessions. We have found that repeated and long (60 minutes) imaginal reliving of the traumatic memory is effective in reducing assault-related symptoms. The procedure called exposure in vivo, or "in real-life," has been found very effective in reducing excessive fears and avoidance after an assault. In this procedure, you will be encouraged to approach safe situations that you have been avoiding since the assault because these situations remind you, directly or indirectly, of the assault (e.g., sleeping with the light off, walking alone in a safe place, or going to a shopping mall).

3. Exposure and Cognitive Restructuring Program

Many survivors of trauma suffer not only from anxiety and avoidance but also from guilt, shame or extreme anger. For those individuals, exposure, described above, with the addition of cognitive restructuring may be the treatment of choice. The three main procedures of this treatment program are prolonged imaginal exposure, in vivo exposure (both described above), and cognitive restructuring. *Cognitive restructuring* aims at teaching you to evaluate how realistic your beliefs are about yourself and the world. After an assault, many assault/rape survivors conclude that the world is unpredictable and uncontrollable, and view the world as entirely dangerous. Another consequence that is common after an assault, is that the survivors develop extremely negative views about themselves. They believe, for example, that the fact that they are experiencing emotional reactions to the trauma indicates that they are less adequate than other people. If you feel this way about yourself, you may have arrived at this common but inaccurate conclusion.

Also, many assault survivors believe that they are extremely vulnerable and incapable of coping with stress. These thoughts cause anxiety, avoidance, and depression and may make PTSD symptoms even worse. A person who is thinking this way may feel anxious much of the time and be less effective in dealing with daily responsibilities. Cognitive restructuring will help you adjust your beliefs and give you skills to realistically evaluate whether a situation is dangerous or not, and whether you are able to cope with it. When you learn to detect these unhelpful thoughts and correct them, your PTSD symptoms should decrease.

Deciding Which Program is for Me

You need to think about the main problems you are experiencing and discuss them with your therapist. Refer back to the description of PTSD symptoms in Chapter 2 and your self-assessment in Chapter 5. Which symptoms are most problematic for you? Are you very avoidant of anything that reminds you of the assault? Is it difficult for you to think about or talk about what happened? Do you not want to go certain places or do things that you used to feel comfortable with? If these are your primary issues to work on, then program 2 should be sufficient to help you.

If you have the above problems but are also very troubled by guilt, shame or extreme anger, program 3, exposure with the addition of cognitive restructuring, may be the treatment of choice. If you are also very aroused and feel out of control and/or don't think you can get yourself to do the imaginal and in vivo exposure, then you may want to start with program 1, SIT. The exposure technique can be added later. We do think it is important for the alleviation of symptoms for those who have been through a trauma to emotionally process the experience. The techniques described above have been shown to be effective in doing this. We recognize that even very effective programs do not work unless the individual is ready to begin. So even if you are not ready at this point, we recommend that you use this program when you are ready to begin.

Obstacles to Change

Let us look at anything that might be an obstacle to your changing. As with any problem, there may be things operating that we cannot easily identify. An example of such an obstacle is the following: if a sick person has been receiving a lot of attention for his/her sickness and/or is excused from chores and duties, there might be some reluctance to get well. Are there things you will be expected to do that you do not want to if your PTSD subsides? Another example is the following: we have seen many women who married men who "came to their rescue" after the assault. In some cases, much of the relationship is built on the partner's protecting and nurturing her. If the woman becomes more independent and stronger, it may require some change in the relationship and this change may be quite threatening to the partner. Obviously, a loving partner wants her to get well and mostly may not be aware of his reluctance to see changes in the relationship, but you should pay attention to these issues or other obstacles to your changing. Often, when one person changes, it changes the relationship. Sometimes such obstacles can be anticipated and dealt with productively by discussing these issues with your partner and therapist.

The following chapter will begin the training in useful techniques with relaxation training.

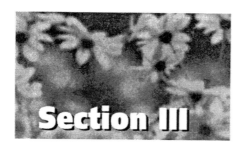

Section III

Cognitive-Behavioral Program

Confronting The Traumatic Memories

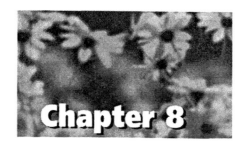

Chapter 8

Relaxation Training: Breathing Retraining, Deep Muscle Relaxation, Differential Relaxation

Breathing Retraining

This chapter will describe breathing retraining and relaxation training. Not everyone will need this in therapy. If you are using the SIT program, it will be helpful to you. If you do not need or already know about this topic, you may skip to the next section. Most of us realize that our breathing affects the way that we feel. For example, when we are upset, people may tell us to take a deep breath and calm down. However, taking a deep breath often does not help. Instead, in order to calm down, one needs to take a normal breath and exhale slowly.

Your therapist will teach you breathing techniques. Here is how it works. First, take in a *normal* breath rather than a deep breath, inhale normally through your nose. Unless we are exercising vigorously, we ought to try to breathe through our noses. After inhaling normally, concentrate on the exhalation and drag it out. While slowly exhaling, say the word *calm* silently to yourself while you are exhaling. Calm is a good word to use because in our culture it is already associated with nice things. If we are upset and someone helps us to 'calm down', usually it is associated with comfort and support. It also sounds nice and can be dragged out to match the long, slow exhalation: c-a-a-a-a-a-l-m.

In addition to concentrating on slow exhalation while saying *Calm* to yourself, you need to slow down your breathing. Very often, when people become frightened or upset, they feel like they need more air and may therefore hyperventilate. Hyperventilation, however does not have a calming effect. In fact it generates anxious feelings. Unless we are preparing for one of the three *F's* (i.e., fight, freeze, flee) in the face of a real danger, we often don't need as much air as we are taking in. When we hyperventilate and take in more air, it signals our bodies to prepare for one of the three *F's* and to keep it fueled with oxygen. This is similar to a runner taking deep breaths to fuel her body with oxygen before a race and continuing to breathe deeply and quickly throughout the race. Usually, when we hyperventilate, though, we are tricking our bodies. What we really need to do is to slow down our breathing and take in *less* air. We do this by pausing between breaths to space them out more. After your slowed exhalation, literally hold your breath for a count of four before you inhale the next breath. Repeat the entire sequence 10 to 15 times, for 10—15 breaths, or until it feels right for you. You can refer to the *Breathing Retraining Outline* (Figure 8.1). You should also practice the breathing retraining at least twice per day, as well as when you are feeling particularly tense or distressed throughout the day. It is a skill that you can know how to do but not be any good at unless you practice.

If you have asthma, you will probably not feel comfortable pausing without air in your lungs. If this is true, take a normal breath, then pause to a count of four, then exhale slowly. This way, you may pause (hold your breath) with air in your lungs. This may be more comfortable for you.

Purpose:

- Slow down breathing

- Decrease amount of oxygen in blood

- With practice, decrease anxiety

Breathing Instructions:

1. Take a normal breath in through your nose with your mouth closed.

2. Exhale slowly with your mouth closed.

3. On exhaling, say the word Calm or Relax very slowly, for example: c-a-a-a-a-a-l-m or r-e-e-e-e-e-l-a-a-a-a-a-x

4. Count slowly to 4 and then take the next inhalation.

5. Practice this exercise several times a day, taking 10 to 15 breaths at each practice.

Figure 8.1. **Breathing Retraining Outline**

Relaxation Training

This technique is called Deep Muscle Relaxation and it is designed to help you manage your anxiety and tension. Your therapist will teach you to sequentially tense and relax various muscles in your body while you pay attention to the feelings associated with tension and relaxation. In addition to learning how to relax, you will also learn how to recognize tension in your muscles. You will be asked to produce tension in your muscles and then release the tension all at once. This allows the muscles to become even more relaxed when you release this tension. It's like a pendulum: if we push it, it will go to the other side, but if we pull it back then let it go, it goes over further. Also, in order to reduce the tension in your muscles, you must first notice it. By tensing/relaxing, tensing/relaxing you will be able to notice the contrast between these two states and will be able to detect the early stages of tension when it is easier to do something about it.

Do you remember what it was like for you when you first learned to ride a bike or drive a stick-shift car? Remember when you were first learning? It was difficult to remember when to do everything and in what order. You had to walk yourself through all the steps very slowly. At first these new tasks didn't feel comfortable to you and you might have felt that you could never learn to drive or ride a bike; but eventually with persistence and practice you mastered these skills, and can probably do them now automatically. Relaxation is a skill that requires practice as do other skills. You can know what to do but not be any good at it unless you practice. If you practice every day you will find that you are able to relax very easily and almost automatically when you say to yourself 'Relax' or 'Calm.'

When you are relaxing or tensing, you may experience some unusual feelings such as a floating sensation, heat in your muscles, tingling in your fingers, or very heavy muscles and limbs. These are signs that your body is beginning to relax and your muscles are loosening up. It is also important that you *go with the process* and that you do not fight what your body may be feeling. However, sometimes it happens that women who have been assaulted have an intrusive thought or an image while they are relaxing. If this happens to you, try to keep your eyes closed, let the thoughts pass through your mind, and refocus on the muscle group. If you are feeling too distressed, open your eyes to orient yourself and then close your eyes again when you are feeling more comfortable.

When you tense and relax each muscle group, it is important that you tense only the muscles that you are focusing on. When you tense them, only tense them to a moderate degree. Don't strain your muscles to the point of discomfort or pain.

Your therapist will review with you the muscle groups that you are going to be tensing and relaxing. See Table 8.1 for the muscle groups list.

Table 8.1. **Muscle Groups List for Deep Muscle Relaxation**

- Clench fists

- Bend hands backward at wrists

- Flex biceps muscles

- Push shoulders back into chair

- Hunch shoulders up towards ears

- Tilt head to left shoulder

- Tilt head to right shoulder

- With head down, tuck chin towards chest

- Press your head back against the chair

- Breathe air in deeply through lungs, and hold for a few seconds

- Tense stomach by contracting muscles as if hit in stomach

- Wrinkle up forehead and brow

- Close eyes tightly

- Open mouth wide

- Purse lips

- Bear down slightly on back teeth

- Tense buttocks

- Arch back

- Stretch out right leg and bend toes back

- Stretch out left leg and bend toes back

- Stretch out right leg and point toes away from body

- Stretch our left leg and point toes away from body

- Curl up toes in shoes

When your body gets relaxed, your mind also gets relaxed. In order to enhance this process, after you have relaxed all major muscle groups, you should imagine a pleasant scene. Just allow yourself to relax as much as you would like and focus on each muscle group. After the completion of each major muscle group (e.g., all neck exercises), do the breathing exercises. Proceed in this manner through all of the muscle groups.

Can you think of a scene that is particularly pleasant for you to imagine? Can you describe that scene?

Some examples of a pleasant scene that others have used include walking or sitting on a beach, sitting in front of a roaring fire, walking through the woods, or listening to music. Please imagine this scene as vividly as possible, bringing in the smells, sounds, colors, and textures that are around you as you imagine it. Stay with that image in your private sanctuary and allow your muscles to go limp and relax. Breathe slowly. This is your time to relax. You will not be hurried. Keep your eyes closed and imagine your pleasant scene. Go to that private sanctuary and see the colors around you, inhale the pleasant scents, listen to the sounds and relax further and further. At the end, count backwards from 4 to 1. On the count of 4, move your legs and your feet. On the count of 3, move your arms and your hands. On the count of 2, move your head and your neck, and on the count of 1, open your eyes, feeling refreshed and relaxed. Take your time opening your eyes, you have been relaxing and there is no need to rush.

How did it feel? Did you have any difficulty with any of the muscle groups? Relaxation can be more easily achieved with closed eyes, but if that makes you very uncomfortable, go ahead and keep them open. Find a quiet place for practicing relaxation exercises. Optimal times during the day to practice relaxation are in the morning before getting out of bed, in the afternoon or upon return from work, in the early evening while relaxing after supper, or at bedtime. Initially, we discourage people from listening to the tape and practicing relaxation before bedtime because you may fall asleep and fail to learn relaxation skills. Once you have learned to relax, you can use this as a strategy to help you get to sleep.

Cue-Controlled Relaxation

Cue-controlled relaxation is another relaxation technique. Cue-controlled relaxation can be used daily to reduce tension in situations that remind you of the assault. When you feel stressed out or anxious, which of your muscles are first affected? This week, pay attention to which muscles in your body feel tense, and use this tension as a cue to use your breathing exercises and relaxation. For example, suppose you had a difficult day at work because you were unable to concentrate and you notice that you are clenching your jaw. This will be your cue to start your breathing exercises and to say your cue word (e.g., 'calm' or 'relax') to help you reduce your tension. Do you notice any muscle group in which there is tension right now, or not as relaxed as the rest? Practice breathing, using your cue word, and allow your muscles to go limp and relax for about 5 minutes.

Differential Muscle Relaxation

There is one more relaxation skill to teach you called differential relaxation. We call it differential relaxation because you will be learning to relax specific muscle groups that are not essential for the activity you engage in when you are tense. You may notice that your muscles are feeling tense much of the day. This is because you are anxious and overly alert a good deal of the day. In actuality, when you engage in various activities, you only need to use those muscle groups directly related to that activity. For example, if you are sitting and watching television there is no need to have tension in the muscles in your face, arms, legs, stomach, and buttocks. However, in order to sit upright you need to slightly tense the muscles in your neck and torso.

Let us run a couple of experiments to demonstrate this principle. First, focus on the amount of tension that you feel in your muscles as you sit in the chair. What muscles are feeling tense right now? What are the essential muscle groups that you need to sit in the chair?

Even when we are using muscles for an activity, we do not need a high degree of tension, say the amount when we are tensing the muscles during deep muscle relaxation. Try to keep the minimal amount of tension required for that activity. Now, try to reduce the degree of tension that you feel in the muscle groups that are not essential for you to sit in the chair, and try to allow the other muscles to relax completely. Do you notice a difference?

Next, write your name on a piece of paper and use only the essential muscles necessary for this activity. What muscles are you able to relax while you are writing? What is the essential muscle group that you need to write your name? Only the muscles in your hand and lower arm are tense when writing. Now, stand up and notice the essential muscles that you need to maintain your balance and posture. What muscles are you able to relax while you are standing there? What are the essential muscle groups that you need to maintain your balance? Only the muscles in your shoulders, back, and legs are tense when you stand. Note that this tension is minimal and it is not necessary to tense other muscles, such as those in your arms, buttocks, or face, to stand.

Now, walk around the room and notice what muscle groups are essential to walk and maintain your balance. It is only necessary to tense the muscles in your shoulders, back, hips, and legs. Note that this tension is minimal and you do not need to tense the muscles in your arms or face, for example, to walk around the room.

The idea is to keep the minimal amount of tension in your muscles to complete whatever activity you are engaging in and to allow the rest of your muscles to relax completely. During daily life, we have a lot of unnecessary tension. For example, when we are driving a car, we need some tension in the muscles of our hands and arms. However, some people report "white knuckling it," especially in traffic. All this does is increase our general level of tension. If you can learn how to let much of this tension go, you can go through life more relaxed and comfortable. Be aware of the tension you carry around with you and work on reducing it.

Remember, in order to be successful in your attempt to relax, you have to practice these relaxation techniques daily for a while. Only after repeated practice will you be able to really use them well when you need them. So, make a time every day for your relaxation. Discuss with your therapist any problems that you may experience while using these relaxation techniques.

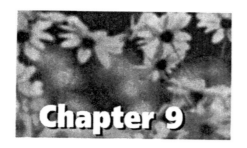

Chapter 9

Real-Life Exposure:
Confrontation of Feared Situations

Feared Situations Hierarchy and Subjective Units of Discomfort Ratings (SUDS)

In this program, we are going to focus on the fears that you are experiencing, and your difficulty coping, both of which are directly related to your assault. By now, you have discussed your thoughts, memories, and emotions concerning the trauma with your therapist. You have also discussed the behaviors, such as avoiding situations and memories that remind you of the assault, that you have been using to reduce the stress associated with thinking about the traumatic event.

A majority of the symptoms experienced after an assault will eventually decline over time. However, some of these problems may not get better on their own in the long run for some survivors. By learning about what causes your symptoms, you can speed up the healing process. Although it is quite normal for people to want to escape or avoid anxiety-provoking and painful emotions, thoughts, and events, doing so actually extends posttrauma reactions. Avoidance provides some short-term relief from distress, but it also prevents you from actually getting over your problems that much sooner.

When you *confront* the painful experiences, you will have the opportunity to process the traumatic event. For example, you don't give yourself a chance to become more comfortable in safe situations if you avoid objectively low-risk assault-related situations. Until you confront your distressing situations, you may keep believing that low-risk situations are dangerous and your anxiety in these situations will never go away. However, by facing these situations, you will find that they are not actually dangerous. Your anxiety and other symptoms will lessen more and more with continual and extended situational confrontations. The same is true for painful memories. Because of this reason, we will ask you to relive the trauma in your imagination over and over (see

Chapter 10) and to confront relatively safe situations that you are now avoiding (in this chapter). This process is what we have referred to as the exposure technique.

In this chapter, we are going to concentrate on your tendency to avoid safe situations and people that are associated with the trauma or remind you of it. In order to help you stop avoiding situations and people that were once enjoyable or important to you, you and your therapist are going to work together to make a list of situations that you have been avoiding since the assault. We call this list "the avoided situation hierarchy," because it is arranged from least distressing to most distressing. To make this list, we want to take into account how much distress or discomfort these situations would cause you if you weren't avoiding them. Therefore we will use a method to indicate your level of distress. Of course we will not ask you to confront unsafe situations. The goal is not to help you view dangerous situations as safe, but rather to help you stop avoiding situations that are realistically quite safe.

Subjective Units of Discomfort

In order to find out how much discomfort certain situations cause you, it is useful for you and your therapist to develop a way to discuss amounts of discomfort. We can do it by imagining that we can measure discomfort on a scale. We call this the SUDS scale which stands for Subjective Units of Discomfort. It's a 0 to 100 scale. A SUDS rating of 100 indicates that you are extremely upset, the most you have ever been in your life, and 0 indicates no discomfort at all. Usually when people say they have a SUDS of 100, they may be experiencing physical reactions, such as sweaty palms, heart palpitations, difficulty breathing, feelings of dizziness, and anxiety. How much discomfort are you feeling now as you are reading? What do you think your SUDS level was during the assault? Remember, the entire scale is measuring discomfort, so even a '10' indicates that you're having some discomfort.

It will be important to become familiar with using the SUDS scale because it is a precise way for you to communicate your feelings with your therapist. You and your therapist will be using SUDS ratings to keep track of your progress during the imaginal and in vivo (in real-life) exposures. It is almost like an anxiety thermometer, you and your therapist will be "taking your anxiety temperature" every few minutes. Increases or decreases in your anxiety level can be detected by using the SUDS method. Almost always, continuing to be exposed to distressful situations results in an eventual reduction in anxiety. This process is called *habituation*. You will find out that even if you are very anxious in certain situations, by staying in them, your anxiety will gradually decrease, indicating that you are habituating.

Following is an example that illustrates how habituation works. A little boy was sitting on the beach with his mother when an unexpected, forceful wave from the ocean washed over them. The child got extremely upset and cried that he wanted to go home. The next day when it was time to go to the beach, the little boy began crying and refused to go. He kept saying "no . . . no . . . water come to me." In order to help him overcome his fear of the water, his mother took him for walks on the beach over the next few days. She would hold his hand and gradually helped him walk closer to the water's edge. After a few days, they played at the water's edge and used water in sand castle building. By the end of the week the boy was able to walk into the water alone. With patience, practice, and encouragement he had habituated to his fear of the water. If he had not been helped to gradually expose himself to being near and in the water, in all likelihood his fear would have remained unchecked, and he would have avoided the water indefinitely. We can get over scary situations if we do it the right way.

Another example is provided by a taxicab driver who lived in New York and who developed a fear of driving across bridges. This fear created serious problems with his work because he was unable to drive customers across bridges. Each time he approached a bridge he pretended that something was mechanically wrong with the taxi and called another cab to take his customers to their destination. The taxicab driver, with the support of a therapist, practiced driving over bridges daily. Within a week's time he was able to go across the bridge with the therapist following him in another car. And in two weeks, with repeated practice, he was able to drive over small bridges by himself.

These are a few examples to help you understand how systematic confrontation with a feared situation can reduce your level of discomfort. Because you have experienced a traumatic event you may need more time to confront fears related to your assault. But with time, practice, and courage you will be able to confront the things that now make you afraid.

Avoided Situation Hierarchy Construction

You and your therapist will use the *Avoided Situation Hierarchy Form* (Figure 9.1) to help develop a list of situations that you are avoiding and to rate the intensity of anxiety you imagine you will have when confronting these situations.

Avoided Situation Hierarchy Form

Name _____

Date _____

Item   **SUDS**

1. _____   _____

2. _____   _____

3. _____   _____

4. _____   _____

5. _____   _____

6. _____   _____

7. _____   _____

8. _____   _____

9. _____   _____

10. _____   _____

11. _____   _____

12. _____   _____

13. _____   _____

14. _____   _____

15. _____   _____

16. _____   _____

Figure 9.1.

If you are having trouble coming up with situations that you are avoiding, here's a list of situations that are typically avoided by assault survivors (Table 9.1).

Table 9.1.	List Of Typically Avoided Situations For Assault Survivors

1. Seeing an unfamiliar man
2. Someone standing close to you
3. Being touched by someone (especially someone unfamiliar)
4. Someone coming up behind you
5. Walking down a street
6. Being alone in your home (day or night)
7. Getting into your car at night
8. Being in a crowded mall or store
9. Talking to men or strangers
10. Being in a car stopped at a stoplight
11. Being in a parking lot
12. Going out at night with friends
13. Reading about an assault in the newspaper or hearing about an assault on television
14. Talking with someone about the assault
15. Seeing the names and pictures of assailants
16. Going to the building or street where you were assaulted
17. Riding public transportation
18. Hugging and kissing significant others
19. Sexual or physical contact
20. Wearing clothes similar to those worn during assault

You do not need to include *every* situation that frightens you or that you avoid on the hierarchy. This is supposed to be a *representative* list to teach you the idea behind exposure therapy—namely, that by repeatedly confronting feared situations that are realistically safe, your anxiety will decrease. You will want to make sure that there are items representing SUDS of 50, 60, 70, 80, 90, and 100 (or thereabouts), as these will be a major focus of treatment.

Avoided Situation Homework Assignments

Review the Avoided Situation Hierarchy list with your therapist and decide together which situations you will confront during homework. Start with situations which you rated as being between 40 and 60 SUDS. By the end of treatment, you should be practicing daily all the situations listed on the hierarchy.

Please refer to the *Model for Gradual In Vivo Exposure* (Table 9.2). In many cases, you will feel more comfortable in certain situations if you are accompanied. We sometimes refer to this person as your "coach." That doesn't mean the coach should push, cajole you or make you feel guilty. She or he should be there to help you feel safer, and can be supportive, too. The coach should *not* be someone who is inconvenienced by your avoidance, and may therefore not have the patience to let you progress at your own pace. The choice of a coach should be discussed between you and your therapist to try to choose a patient, kind, non-judgmental person who will be there to assist you in the way that is best for you.

Table 9.2.	Model for Gradual In Vivo Exposure

Instructions:

Use this example to help you design your in vivo exposure assignments. Remember that it is important for you to remain in the situation for 30 minutes or until there is a 50% decrease in your SUDS. Record your SUDS before and after the exposure using the homework sheet.

Example: Going to shopping mall

1. Coach accompanies you to shopping mall and you walk around the mall together.

2. Coach accompanies you to shopping mall and stays in a specific area of the mall while you walk around alone.

3. Coach accompanies you to shopping mall and stays in a specific area while you walk into some stores alone.

4. Coach drives you to shopping mall and stays in the parking lot while you walk around mall alone.

5. Coach drives you to shopping mall and leaves parking lot for 30 minutes while you walk around the mall alone.

6. You go to shopping mall alone and your coach waits by a telephone in their home.

7. You go to shopping mall alone and don't tell your coach.

Case Example of Hierarchy Construction

Melanie was raped on her college campus while walking home from the library one night, approximately two years prior to entering for treatment. Since that time, in addition to other PTSD symptoms, she avoided many situations. She avoided leaving her dorm room after dark, even accompanied, which extremely restricted her activities. She slept with the light on, much to the annoyance of her roommate. She would not listen to or read anything that referred to a woman being assaulted, even refusing to complete some class assignments. She no longer wore yellow sweaters or Reebok athletic shoes because she was wearing them at the time of the assault. The rationale for in vivo exposure was explained and discussed, and she agreed with its necessity. What follows is the construction of Melanie's personal hierarchy with her therapist. The dialogue is represented with **T** signifying the *Therapist* and **M** signifying *Melanie*:

T: We want to make a list of some of the situations that you avoid since the assault or that you feel very uncomfortable if you find yourself in. The list doesn't have to be exhaustive, just representative. I'll ask you to give each situation a rating on the 0–100 scale of how uncomfortable or scared you think you'd be in that situation, where "0" indicates no anxiety and "100" indicates extreme discomfort, probably how you felt during the assault. It will be our working list, so don't get worried that these ratings are written in stone. Sometimes it's easier to start from the top. What's the worst situation that you now avoid, even though you know that it is probably safe?

M: Uh, that could be several things. I won't go to the library if I can help it. I definitely won't go to the library at night. Actually, I don't like to go anywhere at night. I like to stay in my dorm room with lots of lights on and lots of people around the place. I get pretty scared if there's no one around the dorm.

T: Okay, let's look at these. Those are all very important situations to include on our hierarchy. Out of those, which is the scariest, the one you avoid the most?

M: I guess that would be going to the library. If I can, I do my work on-line or get someone else to check out what I need. I've only been back there one time since the assault, and I freaked out and had to leave without getting my work done. I could never go there at night.

T: So it sounds like going to the library at night would be at the top of the hierarchy. On that 0–100 SUDS scale, how much would you rate going to the library at night?

M: I don't think I could do it. Campus security even tells people now not to walk alone to the library or on campus at night.

T: That's a good point. If it's not a good thing to do, I certainly won't recommend it or put it on the hierarchy. But I find it hard to believe that no one goes to the library at night anymore.

M: Oh, people still go. They just say not to walk alone.

T: Okay, good. So how much would you rate going to the library at night with someone you trust?

M: I'm scared I would freak out again. I'd have to say 100.

T: That's okay, we just need to make the list now. So let's write that down at the top.

T: You also mentioned that you don't leave your dorm at night. Is that right? How much on this 0–100 scale would you rate leaving your dorm at night, say, with someone you trust?

M: That would be pretty scary, too. I've tried that a couple of times, not recently, and I was too scared, so I just stopped doing it. You asked how much? I guess that's pretty close to going to the library at night, let's say 95.

T: Okay, we'll put that down. You also mentioned just going to the library, that you avoid that. How much do you think it would bother you to go to the library during the day with someone else?

M: That's pretty scary, too. I guess I'd say 95.

T: Is it more or less scary than going out at night with people?

M: I guess it's not quite that scary, but it's close. What did I rate going out at night as? 95? Okay, let's say 90 for the library then.

T: Okay, we're moving right along. Let's write that down. You also mentioned not liking to be at the dorm without lots of lights on and people around. Should we put those on our hierarchy, too? How about just having a reading light on? And what about sleeping? Do you sleep with the lights on or off?

M: On. My roommate is really getting sick of it, too. I even bought her one of those eye mask things to wear at night to try to shut the light out, but she says it's uncomfortable.

T: So it sounds like this is a good thing to work on, getting used to fewer lights on and sleeping without any lights on. How much would that bother you, to sleep without any lights on?

M: Oh, my gosh! In the dark? I have a confession: I keep a flashlight in my night table drawer just in case the lights go out. What about that? Do I have to give that up?

T: Does it cause any problems for you?

M: No. Other people I know keep flashlights around, too.

T: Then why don't you keep yours, too. How about sleeping in the dark?

M: Well, I used to before all this and it never bothered me. I used to sleep better, too. I guess I can try it. Let's say 80. And having fewer lights on when we're up probably wouldn't be as bad. Say around 60.

T: You're doing great with this. Let's write those down.

The following hierarchy list (Figure 9.2) represents the situations discussed up to this point.

Avoided Situation Hierarchy Form

Name _Melanie_

Date _5/25/99_

Item		SUDS
1.		
2.		
3.		
4.		
5.		
6.		
7.		
8.		
9.		
10.		
11.	only necessary light on	60
12.		
13.	sleeping in the dark	80
14.	going to the library, day, accompanied	90
15.	going out at night with people	95
16.	going to the library at night with someone	100

Figure 9.2.   **Avoided Situation Hierarchy List Sample**

T: Okay, what else do you avoid?

M: Um, I don't know.

T: Let's think. Are there things that didn't used to bother you before the assault that bother you now?

M: I had trouble doing an assignment the other day because the reading had one scene where a girl was assaulted and I didn't finish reading it and I didn't write the report. I wanted to ask the teacher for help, to tell him why I couldn't do it and ask for another assignment, but I couldn't do that either.

T: Sounds like those would be good things for us to work on. How much would you rate reading about someone being assaulted? In books, newspapers, seeing it on TV? Are all those the same?

M: Yeah, they would all be about the same. I didn't even really try to finish that reading. As soon as I read she was gonna get hurt, I just stopped. I guess if I had finished it, it probably would have been about a 50. I leave when the news comes on TV, too, just in case they'll report a rape. I guess that would be around the same.

T: You're doing a great job here. Let's put those down. Okay, what else?

M: I can't think of anything.

T: I think I remember when you first came in and we were asking you about avoidance that there were certain clothes that you didn't wear anymore. Is that true?

M: Yeah, I guess. The police still have the clothes I was wearing that night. I guess they have them. I don't want them back. Maybe they gave them to my parents, I don't know. But I had on my favorite yellow sweater and Reeboks. My mom, when we were shopping, bought me a pretty yellow sweater but I haven't worn it. I don't want to wear a yellow sweater. I had an old pair of Reeboks, too, that I don't wear anymore. Now I wear Nikes. Is that what you mean?

T: Exactly. Can you see that there's nothing about a yellow sweater or Reeboks that can hurt you? It's just because in your mind they are associated with the assault that you don't want to wear them.

M: Yeah, I see.

T: Good. Let's put them on our list. How much do you think it would bother you to wear a yellow sweater and Reeboks? Are they the same?

M: Yeah, they'd be the same. Let's see . . . wearing a yellow sweater and Reeboks. I just haven't; it probably wouldn't be too bad. Let's say around 50.

T: Okay, do you think that would be easier or more difficult than reading or watching TV about someone getting assaulted?

M: A little harder, but not much.

T: So wearing a yellow sweater and Reeboks would be a little more difficult than reading or watching TV about someone who was assaulted?

M: Yes.

T: Okay. You also mentioned that you wanted to tell your professor what happened to you, why you couldn't do your assignment, but you couldn't. Is that right?

M: Yeah, I couldn't.

T: In general, do you have a hard time talking about what happened to you? Can you tell people you think should know?

M: Well, most people around here already know. It was in the paper, and I was in the hospital for awhile, and you know how people talk. But nobody says anything to me about it, and I never talk about it. It would be hard to talk about it.

T: Are there people you think it would be helpful for you to talk about it with?

M: Sometimes. If I told that teacher, I probably wouldn't have failed that assignment. I've kinda pushed people away, maybe I'm scared they would want to talk about it. I've done that with my sister, we used to talk about everything, but not anymore. Same with my best friend back home. Ever since this happened.

T: Sounds like we should add that to our hierarchy, too. How much do you think it would bother you to talk with your sister or best friend about what happened to you?

M: Um, that would be pretty hard. Say about 80, I think.

T: Okay. Would that be easier or more difficult than sleeping in the dark?

M: Oh, sleeping in the dark would be scarier.

T: Would it be easier or more difficult than turning some lights off, only keeping the necessary lights on?

M: That would be easier. The lights.

T: Okay. Let's put that in the middle then. Talking to your sister and best friend about what happened to you. Would they be the same?

M: Yes, they'd be about the same.

T: What about telling someone like your teacher?

M: Well, I'd be so embarrassed to tell him to his face. I was thinking about writing him a note and telling him. Would that work?

T: Sure. But I think it's important to be able to talk to people to their faces if you want to, but you're going to do that with your sister and best friend, so I think it's okay to write it to your teacher. How much would that bother you?

M: I don't think that would be too bad. Say about a 40.

T: Okay. Let's write all of these down.

Avoided Situation Hierarchy Form

Name *Melanie*

Date *5/25/99*

Item		SUDS
1.		
2.		
3.		
4.		
5.		
6.		
7.		
8.	writing teacher note about assault	40
9.	reading/watching TV about a rape	50
10.	wearing yellow sweater/Reeboks	55
11.	only necessary lights on	60
12.	telling sister/best friend about assault	70
13.	sleeping in the dark	80
14.	going to the library, day, accompanied	90
15.	going out at night with people	95
16.	going to the library at night with someone	100

Figure 9.3.   Avoided Situation Hierarchy List Sample

T: You've done a great job making this hierarchy. I think we have some real important things down here, and all things you can do and all things that I think will free you up a little. I think we have enough to start with now. If other things come up, we can add them to the list. We're going to take it one step at a time.

About In Vivo Exposure Procedure

In vivo exposure, or real life confrontation begins with situations that evoke moderate levels of anxiety (e.g., SUDS=50), and progresses to more fearful situations (e.g., SUDS=100). During the in vivo exposure exercise, you are instructed to remain in the situation for 30 to 45 minutes or until your anxiety decreases considerably.

Aspects of the situations, such as time of day and the people that are present, can be adjusted to achieve the desired level of anxiety during exposure. For example, for Melanie, going to the library during the day with someone would evoke SUDS of 90, but going at night with someone would evoke a SUDS of 100. Another example to demonstrate how the presence of other people can ease someone into a difficult situation involves Belinda, a female physician, who was raped by a male. Belinda reported that she experienced 100 SUDS while conducting physical exams of her male patients, but her SUDS ratings decreased to 60 when a nurse was present during the exams.

When you are practicing in these situations, you may initially experience anxiety symptoms, such as your heart beating rapidly, your palms sweating, feeling faint; you may want to leave the situation immediately. But in order to get over the fear it is important that you remain in the situation until your anxiety decreases. It is very important to remain in the situation until your SUDS decreases by at least 50%. Once your anxiety has decreased at least 50%, then you can stop the exposure and resume other activities. You do not want to experience a sense of relief upon leaving the situation, as that will reinforce the habit to avoid feared but safe circumstances. The desired outcome is to leave feeling relatively comfortable with that situation. *Most importantly, you want to experience habituation ("getting used to it," feeling much less fearful in the situation).* At this point you will have realized that the situation did not lead to any disaster, that nothing bad happened to you, and that anxiety does not stay forever.

If, however, you leave the situation when you are very anxious, you are again convincing yourself that the situation is very dangerous and that something terrible is going to happen to you. And the next time you go into that situation, your level of anxiety will be high again. If you stay in the situation, your anxiety will decrease and eventually you will be able to enter it without fear. The more frequently you practice each situation on your list, the less anxiety you will be experiencing. As a result you will feel less of an urge to avoid situations and people that are now distressing for you.

Please record your SUDS during exposure homework on the *In Vivo Exposure Homework Recording Form* (Figure 9.4).

In Vivo Exposure Homework Recording Form

Date _____

Name _____

Situation Practiced _____

Instructions: Before performing the in vivo exposure, please answer the following questions in the space provided.

1. What is the worst thing that could happen in this situation?

   _____

2. What is the likelihood that this could happen?

   _____

3. Evaluate the evidence for or against the likelihood of this happening.

Against: _____

_____

_____

For: _____

_____

_____

Ratings During In Vivo Exposure

	Time	SUDS
Pre	____	____
Post	____	____

Comments: _____

_____

_____

Figure 9.4.

Here is an example of a completed In Vivo Exposure Homework Recording Form (Figure 9.5).

In Vivo Exposure Homework Recording Form

Date _____5/25/99_____

Name _____Belinda_____

Situation Practiced _____Going to grocery store alone after work (still light)_____

Instructions: Before performing the in vivo exposure, please answer the following questions in the space provided.

1. What is the worst thing that could happen in this situation?

   _____I could get attacked_____

2. What is the likelihood that this could happen?

   _____50%_____

3. Evaluate the evidence for or against the likelihood of this happening.

Against: _____It's light outside; after work is a busy time; it's in a safe area; I've never heard of anyone getting attacked at that grocery store_____

For: _____You never know; if someone wants to hurt me, there's not much I can do to stop them_____

Ratings During In Vivo Exposure

	Time	SUDS
Pre	5:35	60
Post	6:10	30

Comments: _____It was okay. I got my groceries and drove home and I was fine._____

Figure 9.5.   Sample In Vivo Exposure Homework Recording Form

Safety Assessment During In Vivo Exposure Homework Assignment

In designing in vivo exposure homework assignments, it is important to discuss the safety of situations with your therapist. Realistic consideration should be used in deciding which situations are safe for in vivo exposure and which should be avoided. After an assault, it is sometimes difficult to separate our own subjective fears from whether a situation is realistically safe or not. It may help to think of a person you know who is a good judge, not foolhardy, but not afraid of safe situations, to use as your guide in your mind. When trying to decide if a situation is safe, you can then think, "Okay, would (name) think this was an okay thing to do?" We actually try not to think of a black and white, safe vs. dangerous distinction for the world, because so few situations are that easily classified. We think in terms of an acceptable level of risk. There is some risk involved in almost everything we do (for example, people can have accidents in their home or get sick by eating spoiled food), so we like to think in terms of "are we taking a big risk" or "is this an okay thing to do."

Using In Vivo Exposure in Session

Sometimes your in vivo exposure hierarchy includes items that can be accomplished during the therapy session. Examples are exposure situations such as greeting men or making eye contact with them (if there are any men in the clinic or vicinity), lying on one's back with eyes closed, sitting in a waiting room with unfamiliar people, sitting at a table in a cafeteria by oneself, etc. These situations may be first attempted in the therapy session with the therapist's support, if it seems useful. You should then continue to practice that particular exposure for homework. However, the in vivo hierarchy may not include any situations that are easily conducted in session, in which case you will need to work on these as homework. Homework will be decided on by you working with your therapist.

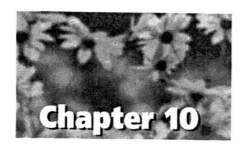

Imaginal Exposure:
Reliving the Trauma Memory in Imagination

Rationale for Imaginal Exposure

In your first session of imaginal exposure, you are going to spend most of the session reliving the memory of your assault in your imagination. It is difficult to understand and make sense of traumatic experiences. When you think about the rape or are reminded of it, you may experience extreme anxiety and other negative feelings such as shame or anger. The assault was a very frightening and distressing experience, so you tend to push away or avoid the painful memories. You may tell yourself, 'Don't think about it; time heals all wounds' or, 'I just have to forget about it.' Other people often advise you to use these same tactics. Also, your friends, family, and partner may feel uncomfortable hearing about the assault, and this may influence you not to talk about it. But, as you have already discovered, no matter how hard you try to push away thoughts about the assault, the experience comes back to haunt you through nightmares, flashbacks, phobias, and distressing thoughts and feelings. These symptoms signal us that your assault is still "unfinished business." In this treatment the goal is to help you process the memories connected with the assault by having you remember them for an extended period of time. Staying with these memories, rather than running away from them, will help decrease the anxiety and fear that are associated with them. It is quite natural to want to avoid painful experiences such as memories, feelings, and situations that remind you of the assault. However, as we already discussed, the more you avoid dealing with the memories, the more they disturb your life. Some of the following examples may help you understand why you need to process the traumatic memories rather than avoiding them.

Imagine that you have eaten a very heavy meal or spoiled food and you now have difficulty digesting it. This can cause you great discomfort, pain, and other symptoms such as fever. But, after you have digested the food you feel a great relief. Similarly, flashbacks, nightmares, and troublesome thoughts are all signs that you have not adequately digested and processed your traumatic experience. With this treatment you are going to start digesting or processing your difficult, heavy memories so that they will stop interfering with your daily life.

Imagine now that your memory is like a very elaborate file cabinet. Past experiences are each filed into a proper drawer. In this way you can organize your experiences and make sense of them. For example, you have a drawer for restaurant experiences. Every time you go to eat in a restaurant you file the memory in this drawer in your mind. This is the way in which you remember how to behave in a restaurant, what to expect and how to evaluate the quality of the food and the services. But in what drawer should you put your assault experience? How should you make sense of it? Part of recovering from a traumatic experience is being able to organize these distressing feelings and memories and find a drawer for them, so you can move on with the business of your life.

Have you ever lost someone that you loved as a result of death or break-up? What was that like for you? Immediately after the loss you may have felt numb, then extremely sad and pained, and you may have also been angry. The way to get over the pain was to experience it, to grieve. After some time, the loss of that person will still be sad, but probably won't cause as intense pain as it used to, and you may be able to think about them without crying. We think this process of grieving is similar to what a person experiences following a trauma. All of these feelings are part of a natural process that an individual may experience after a traumatic event. In fact, it is important to experience all emotions that are connected to a trauma in order to process them and get to a point in which the memories are not so devastating.

The goal of imaginal exposure as well as in vivo (i.e., in real-life) exposure is to begin helping you process the memories associated with your assault by enabling you to have thoughts about the rape, to talk about it or see triggers associated with it without experiencing intense anxiety that disrupts your life. This part of the program includes having you confront situations and memories that generate both anxiety and an urge to avoid. Gradually, the memories will become less painful. You will get used to them. We call this gradual process *habituation*. Repeated reliving of the trauma will also help you in other ways. It will teach you that remembering is not the same as reexperiencing the trauma. In other words, it will help you discriminate between remembering the trauma and being traumatized again. Unlike actually being traumatized again, there is no danger connected with remembering the trauma. Therefore you will learn that you do not need to become overwhelmed with anxiety every time that you think about the rape. Also, repeated reliving will teach you that you are not going to lose control or go crazy if you think about the traumatic memory. On the contrary, through repeated reliving of the rape, you are going to gain control over your memories instead of them having control over you.

And finally, engaging with the traumatic memory repeatedly will allow you to differentiate between the traumatic event and other events that are similar but not dangerous. For example, if now you are afraid of all bald men because you were raped by a bald man, by repeated reliving of the rape you will realize that "baldness" itself is not dangerous.

However, we want to warn you about a common reaction to imaginal exposure: for most people, it will feel as if you are getting worse before you get better. You may experience increased nightmares, anxiety, irritability or intrusive thoughts and this may lead you to want to quit the program. However, this is actually a good sign, although it doesn't feel good. It means you have accessed the memories and are processing them. If you stick with it, it will get better. This just means you've started the process of emotional processing.

The Imaginal Exposure Procedure: How to Practice it

The following section will be described with the assumption that you are working with a therapist. If you are not, read the section and adapt it for work on your own.

Your therapist will ask you to recall the memories of the assault. It is best for you to close your eyes so you won't be distracted, so that you can envision these events in your mind's eye. Your therapist will ask you to recall these painful memories as vividly as possible. We call this reliving. Don't tell a story about the assault in the past tense, but describe the assault in the present tense, as if it were happening now, right here. Your therapist will ask you to close your eyes and tell him or her what happened during the assault in as much detail as you remember. You will work on this together. Remember that you are in a safe room with your therapist. If you start to feel too uncomfortable and want to run away or avoid it by leaving the image, your therapist will help you to stay with it. You will audiotape the narrative so you can take the tape home and listen to it for homework, practicing the imaginal exposure at home. From time to time, while you are reliving the assault, your therapist will ask you for your anxiety level on the 0 to 100 SUDS scale, in which "0" indicates no anxiety or discomfort and "100" indicates panic-level anxiety. Please answer quickly and don't leave the image. The rating should indicate how anxious you are at the time, sitting in the office, not how you felt during the assault. An example of this process follows.

Case Example 1: Emily

Emily was raped in her apartment on a Wednesday night. She had run out to the grocery store after work. She had returned home, put her groceries away, and encountered an intruder. Her imaginal exposure transcript:

I'm in my kitchen. . . and I hear a noise. . . and I turn around expecting to see the cat that I think just jumped up on the counter and instead I see this man. . . and I can't believe it. . . and he's looking at me. . . and he's. . . coming towards me. . . with his hands out like. . . telling me not to scream and he won't hurt me. . . and I'm begging with him not to hurt me. . . and he just keeps saying don't scream and I won't hurt you.. back and forth we keep this up and he tells me to go to the bedroom and sit on the bed. I'm sitting on the edge of the bed. . . thinking. . . who is this man. . . and thinking. . . it's impossible he is in my house. . . I was just gone for several minutes. . . that's about all I feel. . . I'm scared. . . I'm just feeling scared. . . and I'm just shaking. . . and I'm holding on to my can of soda. . . as tight as I can. . . and he makes me lay back. . . I lay back on my bed. . . and I'm staring at the ceiling and he takes the can out of my hand and he puts it down. . . and I'm hearing him do something and I turn my head to the right and I see his penis out of his pants. . . and I'm shocked. . . I never expected to see that. . . and he's telling me to touch it. . . it seemed like a long time passed and I cannot move my hand. And now. . . and now he's moving my hand. . . and. . . he throws off my hand. . . because he is frustrated. And he comes around to the other side of the bed and he's kneeling down. . . and it's like this is just happening to me but I'm not thinking. . . I'm not wondering what he's doing. . . it's just happening. . . one right after another. . . until I feel his mouth on my vaginal area and I'm beginning to just. . . I'm just talking to myself and I'm telling myself it will be okay. . . just let me get through this alive. . . this is not happening. . . and then he's standing up but kind of toward me. . . like leaning on me. . . and my thoughts are what is he doing now. . . I'm sensing that he's having trouble doing whatever he's doing. . . I'm not real sure. . . until I can feel that he just begins to rape me. . . and he's coming towards me and he's kissing me on my lips. . . and he's just sloppy. . . and he smells. . . like alcohol and sweat. . . and I just. . . I'm almost playing dead. . . and then he lowers down and pulls my bra over and he's just kind of slobbering on me. . . and my eyes are shut. . . and my ears are ringing. . . and then he leans up and he says. . . tell me you love me . . . and he's kind of saying in a real harsh voice. . . and I'm telling myself. . . don't do it. . . and he's saying it again. . . and he's getting

mad. . . he's repeating again and again tell me you love me. . .
and I quick respond yes. . . I'm more angry at him asking me
to tell him I love him than I am about him raping me. . . cause
before I could pretend that this just wasn't happening but now
I am mad. . .I'm feeling mad. . . I'm feeling like I'm being
forced to say yes. . . and I continue to stare at him. . . and he's
so scary I start to cry and I'm asking him why he's doing this to
me. . . he just gets up. . . stops raping me. . . I'm sitting up. . .
and he says have you got any money. . . and I say yes. . . and
then I turn over looking for my purse and I find five dollars. . .
and I give it to him. . . and he's telling me to stay in the
bedroom and lock the door. . . so I just respond. . . and while
I'm sitting in my bedroom I'm hearing him on the other side
of the door. . . and I shake more. . . all over. . . I cannot control
it. . . I'm so scared that he's coming again. . .. and then I don't
hear him anymore so I sit there and just stare at the wall. . .
and after about 10 minutes I get up and run through the living
room and leap down the steps and run across to my neighbors
and ring the doorbell repeatedly until my neighbor answers
the door. . . and she has this look of shock on her face. . . and
I quickly say I've just been raped and she lets me inside. . . I'm
in shock. . . I can't think what just happened. . . and I'm afraid
that he's still close by and can get to me. . . I'm scared. . . it's
as if I have no control in my life cause I won't stop shaking. . .
no matter what I do. . . my whole body . . . it won't stop
shaking. . . and then I just call the police and then it's just. . .
so disorganized. . . just. . . police arrive. . . I'm not looking
around. . . I'm just staring at my legs. . . my feet. . . and part of
me is very relieved. . . the police keep saying I don't have to go
to the hospital. . . I don't have to cooperate. . . I don't have to
tell them anything. . . I just keep telling them whatever it takes
to get him caught. . . I'll do whatever it takes to get him
caught. . . I just can't say that enough to them. . . I'm crying
almost the whole time I'm at my neighbors. . . I finally calm
down when the ambulance gets there. . .I'm feeling calm
when the ambulance gets there. . .and I am stepping into
the ambulance all by myself. . .I'm not sure what is happening
. . .and there is police just going all over the place. . .I'm
cold. . .I'm shaking, cold. . . Numb. . . I'm in shock. . .I don't cry
anymore, I just stare out the back window of the ambulance
the entire drive . . .and I can hear the people in the ambulance
telling me to relax. . . just feel. . .numb.

Emily described feeling emotionally numb at times during and after her
assault. This is a reaction she described during her imaginal exposure, as well.
In later sessions, her therapist worked on helping Emily to feel all of the

emotions associated with her assault while reliving it to aid in her emotional processing of this trauma.

Sometimes clients are frightened of what they may remember during imaginal exposure. Whatever you remember, it does not change what happened: that you survived, and that you did the right thing for survival. We have not yet encountered a client who remembered details during imaginal exposure that she could not cope with. One of our patients described each session of exposure therapy as "peeling a layer off of an onion, and after a few sessions, you get to the stinky part in the middle, and then it doesn't stink anymore."

After the reliving, think about your reactions. Was it as bad as you thought it would be? You should be very proud of yourself; it takes courage to do what you are doing. You'll need to listen to the tape of your imaginal reliving at home to continue to practice. Try to close your eyes and practice the imaginal exposure at home like you did in session, really seeing it, rather than just listening to a tape. Is there a private place where you can listen to the tape where no one else can hear or will disturb you? Portable tape players with earphones are useful for privacy. We don't encourage letting significant others listen to the tapes for various reasons. One, we don't want you monitoring what you say thinking about an audience, and two, it may be very upsetting for other people to hear with no therapist present to help them. In unusual circumstances, though, it is allowed. Remember to record your anxiety level and any comments each time you practice on the Exposure Homework Recording Form (Figure 10.1).

Exposure Homework Recording Form

Name _____ Date _____

Description of exposure in imagination _____

_____

Date _____

Pre Imaginal Exposure SUDS   _____

Post Imaginal Exposure SUDS   _____

Comments _____

Date _____

Pre Imaginal Exposure SUDS   _____

Post Imaginal Exposure SUDS   _____

Comments _____

Date _____

Pre Imaginal Exposure SUDS   _____

Post Imaginal Exposure SUDS   _____

Comments _____

Date _____

Pre Imaginal Exposure SUDS   _____

Post Imaginal Exposure SUDS   _____

Comments _____

Date _____

Pre Imaginal Exposure SUDS   _____

Post Imaginal Exposure SUDS   _____

Comments _____

Figure 10.1.

Here is an example of a completed Exposure Homework Recording Form:
(Figure 10.2)

Exposure Homework Recording Form

Name *Emily*   Date   *5/29/99*

Description of exposure in imagination *Description of exposure in imagination the*
assailant in my apartment, the assault, and immediately afterwards

Date *5/29/99*

Pre Imaginal Exposure SUDS   *50*

Post Imaginal Exposure SUDS   *40*

Comments *not too bad*

Date *5/30/99*

Pre Imaginal Exposure SUDS   *40*

Post Imaginal Exposure SUDS   *30*

Comments *getting easier*

Date *5/31/99*

Pre Imaginal Exposure SUDS   *40*

Post Imaginal Exposure SUDS   *30*

Comments *about the same*

Date _____

Pre Imaginal Exposure SUDS   _____

Post Imaginal Exposure SUDS   _____

Comments _____

Figure 10.2.   Sample Exposure Homework Recording Form

Following is a description of treatment that incorporates imaginal exposure. It
contains excerpts of an actual exposure session, with comments about what
is going on, and is reprinted from Rothbaum and Foa (1992).

Case Example 2: Susan

Susan was a 31-year-old married white woman in graduate school. She was upstairs in her townhouse studying for a test when her husband left to make a quick trip to the store. A black man in his 20's entered her house, robbed her, and raped her at what she thought was knifepoint. She was hit and threatened when she screamed. After the rape was completed and the rapist was adjusting his clothing, Susan made a dash for the door and was caught in a struggle, but managed to escape.

Susan entered for treatment approximately one year following this incident complaining of nightmares, fears of being alone, avoidance of sex with her husband, hypervigilance, jumpiness, and decreased concentration and consequent difficulties in school. She reported avoiding taking the dog for walks after dark, avoiding being downstairs in her house when alone, constantly checking locks, and avoiding discussing the assault. Treatment consisted of prolonged imaginal exposure as described above and self in vivo exposure as homework.

Susan responded well to treatment. She complied with treatment instructions in carrying out all exposures despite high anxiety. Her anxiety decreased both within sessions and between sessions as indicated by her SUDS ratings and observable discomfort. She maintained treatment gains at follow-up assessments 3, 6 and 12 months after treatment, and became highly functional as reflected by her professional and family achievements.

Session excerpts

> . . . I see this person in the doorway of the stairwell and he seems to be rushing at me. . . And my heart's pounding. . . I'm really surprised. . . and I know I'm really in trouble. . . He has this thing at my head and he says if you scream, which I don't cause I got fingers practically down my throat. . . that he'll shoot me . . .

In this excerpt, Susan describes the scene in the present tense. She has included physical reactions ("my heart's pounding"), meaning appraisals ("I know I'm really in trouble"), threat ("he'll shoot me"), and detailed stimuli and action. The inclusion of all these stimuli and response elements in imaginal exposure scenarios has been found to help the activation of the fear structure. When only stimuli were described (and not responses), less fear responses have been observed. Enhanced activation of fear has been found to be positively related to treatment gains.

> . . . he says, 'Where did your husband go?' and I say, 'Just out
> to do something very quickly, he'll be right back.' And he says,
> 'I've got my buddy waiting for him.' And that really scares me
> because it seems like now this is some type of horror story or
> something. . . that we're both going to be hurt. . .

Here, the assailant makes a threat that extends into the future and involves her husband. Now, Susan's trauma has been broadened and she is in the position of considering the future consequences of her actions as well as the safety of her husband.

> . . . he says, 'Get on the bed,' which again surprises me. . .
> I didn't expect that. . . it's the first time I suspect rape. . .
> So I get on the bed. . . I don't see any choice, any way to
> escape. . . I think there is somebody downstairs. . .

When confronted with an intruder, many survivors report that they were surprised when they realized they were going to be raped and not just robbed. Experts think that unpredictability ("I didn't expect that") and uncontrollability ("I don't see any choice, any way to escape") are related to the development of PTSD. The fight for control is expressed in the following excerpt.

> . . . he whacks me across the face. . . and he says "don't scream
> anymore". . . I think this man is really dangerous, he really can
> hurt me and I have to be careful, so I have to figure out how
> much anything I try to do is going to provoke him and not let
> it get that far.

Susan's attempts to call for help through screaming are punished which prompts her to try different strategies. Many survivors become passive during the assault, which may help them to survive by not provoking their assailant especially when a weapon is present. No one is prepared to confront a rapist, and therefore the response of the victim during the rape relies totally on momentary improvisation.

> . . .he's pushing too low and I feel burning, sharp, cutting and
> then it goes in. . . and I don't really feel it after that, just like
> movement. . . he says, "When I'm done with you. . . my buddy's
> coming up,". . . that's just another terrifying moment. . . I want
> to get out, I can't have that. . . another person. . . going to hit
> me. . . I'm saying, "No, no, please don't hurt me, no, no,". . .
> and I hate it, I hate whining. I hear myself saying it and I wish
> I would stop, it's like I can't make myself stop. . .

Susan is describing some dissociative reactions, which are very common at the time of the assault. Susan's dissociative responses are minimal ("I don't really feel it after that. . .I hear myself saying it"), but more blatant dissociation is common among rape survivors. This may include a sense of "leaving one's body and watching the assault as an outsider." An extreme dissociative reaction involves psychogenic amnesia (inability to recall important aspects of the situation). In these cases, imaginal exposure has been found helpful in aiding recall of details that were previously not recalled. For example, during the third session of imaginal exposure, one patient recalled for the first time that her assailant cocked the pistol he was holding to her head and threatened to pull the trigger if she did not perform fellatio. Thereafter, she was able to describe her assault in more detail and within six sessions her fear dissipated. This integration of previously dissociated detail appears to facilitate recovery.

> . . . he comes off of me, says. . . "Kiss it," which I don't wanna do. . . my mouth's bleeding and it hurts. . . it just looks evil and I think it's dirty. . . and I don't want to do it, but he pushes me down and I'm afraid I'm going to be hurt. . . so I just do it. . .

Susan is again describing a perceived lack of control and a fear of further injury. In this particular session, she did not describe the fellatio in detail. In subsequent sessions, however, she had included a detailed description of the assault including her responses. It is important to include all memories, including olfactory (smell), visual (seeing), auditory (hearing), and tactile (touch). The integration of detail from different sensory modalities facilitates recovery, as these details, when left fragmented, can act as seemingly random event triggers of fear.

> . . . I'm shaking now, it's cold,. . . and I'm embarrassed. . . It's very peculiar. . . it's like I'm again suspended, and I'm nude in my bedroom with someone I don't know. . . it's like this same feeling when you dream that you're at work, but you're not dressed correctly, like you wore your pajamas to work or something. . . sort of a little panic and embarrassed and you don't want anyone to see you. . .

This is a rich description of the feelings that might arise during the assault. The embarrassment and shame Susan described is common in rape survivors and likely inhibits disclosure which may hinder emotional processing.

Outline of Treatment Sessions

Now that you have read about some of the methods by which Cognitive-Behavioral Therapy helps you in recovering from PTSD, you may want to know how these methods fit within the structure of your therapy sessions. If you are in therapy with a therapist following this program, the outline below suggests how your sessions might be organized. Be sure and consult with your therapist about this, as the sequence may vary to suit your individual treatment needs.

Session 1 Outline

A. Your therapist will most likely describe this program and the treatment procedures that will be used in the program, discuss your PTSD symptoms and ask you to read the Rationale for Treatment section of your workbook.

B. Your therapist will probably collect information about your assault

C. Your therapist may teach you breathing retraining at this time (see Chapter 8 for instructions)

D. You will have the following homework to complete before each session:

1. Practice breathing retraining for 10 minutes, 3 times a day

2. Read the Rationale for Treatment section (Chapter 10) of your workbook and note questions

Session 2 Outline

A. Your therapist may discuss the Common Reactions to Assault (See Chapter 4)

B. You may discuss the rationale for the treatment program in detail

C. You may prepare for in vivo exposure (see Chapter 9) by training in SUDS, constructing the avoided situation hierarchy, and selecting your in vivo assignments to practice for homework

D. You may have the following homework to complete before your next session:

1. Read Common Reactions to Assault chapter daily

2. Continue to practice breathing retraining

3. Review the list of avoided situations at home and add additional situations

4. Begin in vivo exposure assignments

Session 3 Outline

A. You may prepare for imaginal exposure by discussing the rationale

B. You may engage in imaginal exposure

C   You may have the following homework to complete before your next session:

    1. Continue breathing practice

    2. Listen to audiotape of imaginal exposure at least once a day.

    3. Continue with in vivo exposure exercises daily working up the hierarchy with SUDS levels.

Sessions 4–7 Outline

A. Imaginal exposure

B. In vivo exposure (discussion and/or practice)

C. You will most likely have the following homework to complete before your next session:

    1. Continue breathing practice

    2. Listen to imaginal exposure tape daily

    3. Continue to perform in vivo exposure exercises

Session 8 Outline

A. Imaginal exposure

B. In vivo exposure (discussion and/or practice)

C. You and your therapist may at this time evaluate your progress in treatment and decide the number of sessions remaining

D. You may have the following homework to complete before your next session:

    1. Continue breathing practice

    2. Listen to imaginal exposure tape daily

    3. Continue to perform in vivo exposure exercises

Session 9 (Only If *Not* the Final Session), Sessions 10–11 Outline

A. Imaginal exposure

B. In vivo exposure (discussion and/or practice)

C. You may have the following homework to complete before your next session:

    1. Continue breathing practice

    2. Listen to imaginal exposure tape daily

    3. Continue to perform in vivo exposure exercises

Session 12 (Final Session) Outline

A. Imaginal exposure

B. In vivo exposure (discussion and/or practice)

C. Review your progress with your therapist and discuss continued practice

D. Terminate therapy: saying good-bye to your therapist

Additional Reading

Rothbaum, B. O., & Foa, E. B. (1992). Exposure therapy for rape survivors with post-traumatic stress disorder. *The Behavior Therapist*, October, 219-222.

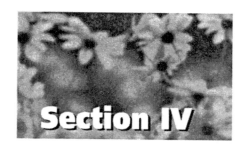

Cognitive-Behavioral Program

Stress Management Techniques

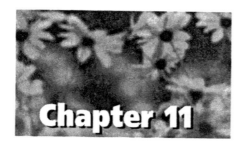

Chapter 11

Cognitive Techniques I: Cognitive Restructuring

Rationale For Cognitive Therapy

Below is a description of why cognitive therapy is helpful in dealing with the psychological aftermath of assault. This explanation is also provided in *Treating the Trauma of Rape: Cognitive-Behavioral Therapy for PTSD*.

After an assault, which is an extremely traumatic event, our thoughts and beliefs about ourselves and the world can undergo a drastic change. Often survivors believe that the world is extremely dangerous and that they are unworthy people who cannot cope. The goal of treatment is to help you evaluate your thoughts and beliefs about safety and your thoughts about yourself, and it is important to identify the unhelpful beliefs that make you feel distressed and prolong your PTSD symptoms.

Let's discuss an example. Before the assault, you may have felt that the world was a safe place and that you were able to handle challenging situations. Many women tell us that after an assault they feel anxious about, and afraid of many things, including: being alone at home, going to work, going shopping, or being with a man. Have you had similar experiences? When you experienced these feelings, did you notice what you were saying to yourself?

After you were assaulted, you may have started to think that almost every place in your world is dangerous. Is this a rational thought? Obviously the world is not entirely safe, otherwise you would not have been assaulted. So how should one evaluate safety? To answer this question, it will help to imagine that there is a range of beliefs about world safety, with a belief that the world is extremely safe on one end and a belief that the world is extremely dangerous on the other end. We have found that the most rational beliefs are somewhere in the middle of this continuum. This assumption is based on the lives of most people in our society and on the fact that safety varies with life circumstances. Understanding safety as a continuum in which safety may vary across different circumstances allows us to evaluate the relative safety of our life circumstances. Viewing safety on a continuum allows us to recognize that many situations are quite safe such as going to work, leaving your house, walking down the street, or spending time with people. On the other hand, in reality, there *are* situations where you need to use your safety guidelines. There are certain places or situations where you should not be alone or be trusting. For example, a woman should not be walking alone late at night in a high-crime area. Awareness of your environment and using good judgement are always a good idea. However, this does not mean that the entire world is an unsafe place and that you cannot conduct your life with some sense of freedom and safety. A better ability to distinguish safe from unsafe places allows you to be better prepared to handle unsafe places and to relax in places that are safe.

After a traumatic event, many women see the world as completely dangerous and begin avoiding many safe situations and people. The belief that the world is a dangerous place naturally leads to PTSD symptoms such as general anxiety, hypervigilance (constantly being on the lookout for any sign of potential danger in the world around you) and unnecessary avoidance of situations. Do you now have the sense that a lot of situations are not safe?

One reason for having a pervasive sense of danger following an assault may be that the assault occurred in a place previously seen as safe, such as one's home. In this case, it is important to understand specifically what may have allowed the place to be violated.

In addition to thinking that the world is a dangerous place, many assault survivors feel that they are "not in control" and think that they are incompetent and cannot cope with stress. For example, after an assault a woman who was able to handle the daily demands of her children now finds that with increased stress she is extremely irritable and unable to handle daily problems. This type of experience creates a domino effect that can lead her to believe that she is unable to cope with normal demands, that she is not a good mother, or that she is losing control. These feelings and thoughts, that she is unable to cope, bring on an overall feeling of lack of control and incompetence. Also, there can be an increase in the feelings that the person is in constant danger. Do you experience similar thoughts about yourself?

Another common belief after a trauma is that the common reactions to trauma which we have discussed before such as intrusive thoughts, flashbacks, and nightmares are signs that something is wrong with you as a person and are taken as evidence of going crazy. This idea leads you to try to suppress recollections and thoughts about the trauma. Paradoxically, however, the more you try to push these thoughts away, the stronger they become and the less control you have over them. In this way, attempts to suppress thoughts about the trauma actually increase the PTSD symptoms. Do you find yourself working hard to not think about your rape?

What is Cognitive Restructuring?

The aim of cognitive restructuring is to identify, challenge, and modify the unhelpful beliefs that cause you intense anxiety, guilt, anger or sadness. Automatic thoughts (ATs) occur automatically (hence the name) and are not deliberate thoughts. They are brief and discrete statements that people say to themselves. Automatic thoughts occur near or just below the threshold of our awareness. We are frequently unaware of the fact that we are having these thoughts. Often we are aware only of uncomfortable feelings that seem to come out of nowhere. Sometimes they take the form of underlying beliefs that are not conscious thoughts but influence us greatly.

Overview of Steps for Cognitive Restructuring

1. Identify the situation that caused you emotional distress (e.g., "I was in the mall when I saw this man looking at me.")

2. Identify the emotions you had in the situation (anxious, anger, guilt/shame, sadness)

3. Identify the thoughts that caused the emotion (e.g., "He is looking at me in a funny way.")

4. Identify beliefs that underlie the thought by continuing to ask yourself the question, "So what does this mean that he looks at you in a funny way?" (e.g., "He is going to hurt me.")

5. Challenge the belief by collecting evidence to support or refute it

6. If insufficient evidence exists to support the belief, continue by asking questions that aim to modify the belief

7. If sufficient evidence exists to support the belief, restate the belief rationally and adaptively or seek a safety response (e.g., "It is not safe to walk in my neighborhood at night. There are drug pushers on every corner. I should go out only with other people that I can trust.")

Rationale for Cognitive Restructuring

The skill that you are going to learn here and with your therapist is to identify the negative thoughts that are causing you to feel very anxious or distressed. This is because these thoughts interfere with your functioning. Many times negative thoughts are not based on reality or fact. These thoughts come into our minds so quickly that sometimes we aren't even aware that we are having them. We are responding to an automatic thought when we realize something has "pushed our button" and we overreacted.

These thoughts are problematic because they lead to excessive or unrealistic negative emotions such as anxiety, anger, guilt or sadness. We would like to help you become aware of these distressing and uncomfortable thoughts and then consider whether they are helpful or not. We are going to work together on trying to identify your unhelpful thoughts and beliefs and then discuss them in a more objective way.

One way to become more objective is to pretend that we are scientists or detectives who develop hypotheses and collect evidence to negate or support these hypotheses/beliefs. Therefore, as we investigate and look for evidence, we need to be objective and attempt to separate feelings from fact or reality.

Identification of Negative Thoughts and Beliefs

The purpose of cognitive restructuring is to teach you to identify key *thoughts or beliefs* that make you feel upset. Anger, guilt, fear, or sadness are examples of *feelings*. When people are upset it is because they are saying something to themselves. Your therapist is going to teach you a method to manage your distressing thoughts and feelings. He or she will teach you how to examine your thinking to objectively evaluate the accuracy of the thoughts or beliefs that cause you distress. You will also learn to evaluate where you might be jumping to conclusions or blowing things out of proportion.

The following are examples of non-assault and assault-related situations that often lead to automatic thoughts:

Non-assault-Related Examples

- A co-worker that doesn't say hello to you in the morning
- Going for a job interview
- Getting a parking ticket

- Going out on a date
- Going to the grocery store at night
- An argument with a friend or significant other
- Talking with a man

Three Important Points About Automatic Thoughts

1. Automatic thoughts occur automatically and are *not* intentional. Instead, they are brief, discrete statements that people say to themselves. The result of these statements can be distress. Frequently we are not aware that we are having these thoughts or uncomfortable feelings.

2. Just because we have these thoughts does not mean that they are true. For example, one may have a thought that "the world is flat" but that does not mean that it is really flat.

3. Negative thoughts are often difficult to identify because they are habitual and rapid. Troublesome thoughts of the assault/rape and visual images play a major role in the feelings that you are experiencing. The images that are associated with the assault/rape can be embarrassing or produce guilt feelings. It may be difficult for you to discuss these thoughts. You may feel that the only way to cope with these distressing thoughts is to avoid thinking about them and distract yourself. But in order for you to be able to challenge and evaluate these thoughts, you have to take a good long look at them.

Challenging Negative Thoughts

After you have identified your negative thoughts, you need to learn how to *challenge* these thoughts and replace them with more helpful rational thoughts or beliefs. This is accomplished by asking questions about the meaning and accuracy or validity of these thoughts. This process is not the same as "the power of positive thinking." The purpose is not to trade negative thoughts for positive ones. Rather, the goal of challenging the dysfunctional negative thoughts is to recognize the errors in one's logic and thinking that cause distress. We will discuss below how thoughts that are strongly charged with emotion are more likely to be general, absolute, and consequently less objective. Therefore, these errors need to be corrected and exchanged for thoughts that are objective, reasonable, and that more accurately reflect reality. See Figure 11.1.

The goal of cognitive restructuring is to help you think and react more objectively, and to respond logically rather than emotionally. Common cognitive errors include: assuming danger when none is present, feeling degraded and/or guilty because one has been raped, assuming all men are rapists, thinking people cannot be trusted, and feeling rejected easily. To really change one's thinking is a slow process. The work during the therapy sessions is just the beginning; you must practice this disciplined type of thinking at every opportunity. If you do, the new thinking habits will become automatic and you should feel much more emotionally stable, and less like an emotional roller coaster.

Challenges to Negative Thought

1. What evidence do I have for this thought? _____
    _____

2. Is there any alternative way of looking at the situation? _____
    _____

3. Is there any alternative explanation? _____
    _____

4. How would someone else think about the situation? _____
    _____

5. Are my judgments based on how I felt rather than what I did? _____
    _____

6. Am I setting for myself an unrealistic and unobtainable standard? _____
    _____

7. Am I forgetting relevant facts or focusing too much on irrelevant facts? _____
    _____

8. Is this an example of all-or-nothing or black and white thinking? _____
    _____

9. Am I overestimating how much control and responsibility I have in this situation? ____
    _____

10. What would be the worst thing that could happen? _____
    _____

11. If this is true, what does that mean, or so what? What would be so bad about that? ____
    _____

12. How will things look, seem, or work in X (number) months? _____
    _____

13. What are the real and probable consequences of the situation? _____
    _____

14. Am I underestimating what I can do to deal with the problem or situation? ____
    _____

15. Am I confusing a low-probability event with one of high probability? _____
    _____

16. Where is the logic in this thought? _____
    _____

17. What are the advantages and disadvantages of thinking this way? _____
    _____

Figure 11.1.

Common Cognitive Distortions

Cognitive distortions are errors in thinking that trigger negative thoughts and beliefs, which in turn trigger negative emotions. We're going to review a list of common cognitive distortions that people make. The following list is similar to cognitive distortions discussed by Burns (1980). Think about these cognitive distortions and see if you can identify which patterns of negative thought you use often.

Examples of Cognitive Distortions

1. *All or Nothing Thinking*: You see the world as black or white, or you fit information into all or nothing categories. For example, if your performance falls short of perfect, you see yourself as a failure. Another example of this is that the world is either completely safe or totally dangerous. Are you aware of all or nothing thinking?

2. *Overgeneralization*: You see a single negative event as a never-ending pattern. You may arbitrarily conclude that a single negative event will happen again and again. An example of this is the thought "I am going to be raped again." or "Bad things keep happening to me so I must be a bad person." Do you tend to overgeneralize? Do you have a personal example?

3. *Must, Should, or Never Statements*: These are unwritten rules or expectations for your behavior that are based on myths or rules rather than facts. These distortions can create feelings of discomfort, anxiety, fear, sadness, or anger. They are inflexible rules for your behavior that you learned when you were growing up, which create expectations that you must live up to. Some examples of these statements are "I should be able to handle this" or "I never should have fought back" or "I should have fought off my assailant." Can you think of any must, should, or never statements that you say to yourself?

4. *Catastrophizing*: This type of distortion happens when you focus on the most extreme negative consequences. This leads to heightened fear and anxiety. You may expect disaster to happen. Most catastrophizing thoughts are triggered by *"what if"* thoughts such as "What if I were in the bathroom and someone came in?" or "What if I were being followed by the man in the grocery store?" An example of this would be one of the following: "If this light doesn't turn green, I am going to go crazy and lose control" or "If this man doesn't stop following me, I am going to be assaulted." Can you think of any catastrophizing statements that you say?

5. *Emotional Reasoning*: This type of distortion arises when what you feel determines what you think. While it is important to pay attention to how you feel, your feelings can lie to you. In fact, if you are anxious most of the time your feelings are almost certainly lying to you. An example of emotional reasoning would be one of the following: "I am very nervous around men, therefore they must want to hurt me" or "I feel very anxious in this situation, therefore I am going to go crazy and lose control" or "Since I feel afraid, there must be something to be scared of" or "I feel panic, the world must be dangerous." These thoughts are emotion driven. Can you think of an example of this in your own life?

Demonstration of Using the Daily Diary

You have begun the first step towards identifying and challenging your distressing feelings and thoughts. Over the next few days, it would be helpful if you kept a diary about some of the situations, thoughts, and feelings that you experience (positive or negative) using this diary form (Figure 11.2). A sample diary entry can be found in Figure 11.3. Try to record in your diary at least 3 times a day between now and your next session with your therapist. Also, read the above Examples of Cognitive Distortions list several times until you become familiar with the distortions. Use it to identify the distortions that you find yourself making as you record in your diary. Bring this daily diary to your therapy session each time for you and your therapist to work on.

Daily Diary

Date _____

1. Situations	3. Negative Thoughts	4. Challenge to Negative Thoughts	5. Rational Response
Describe: 1. Actual event leading to unpleasant emotion or 2. Thoughts or recollections leading to unpleasant emotion	1. Write automatic thought(s) that preceded emotion(s) 2. Rate belief in automatic thought(s) 0–100%. Specify:	Use the questions on the back of this page to challenge negative thought. For instance, list evidence for and against the thought here. Evidence For: Evidence Against:	1. Write rational response to automatic thought(s) 2. Rate belief in rational response 0–100
2. Emotions 1. Sad/anxious/angry, etc. 2. Intensity of emotion 1–100			

Figure 11.2.

Daily Diary

Date _____

1. Situations	3. Negative Thoughts	4. Challenge to Negative Thoughts	5. Rational Response
Describe: 1. Actual event leading to unpleasant emotion or 2. Thoughts or recollections leading to unpleasant emotion *Saw man in mall who looked like the assailant* **2. Emotions** 1. Sad/anxious/angry, etc. 2. Intensity of emotion 1–100 *anxious 90* *panicky 90*	1. Write automatic thought(s) that preceded emotion(s) 2. Rate belief in automatic thought(s) 0–100%. Specify: *He's going to hurt me/I'm in danger* *80%*	Use the questions on the back of this page to challenge negative thought. For instance, list evidence for and against the thought here. Evidence For: *—He's dressed like the assailant (baggy pants, tennis shoes)* *—He's about the same age* *—He's the same race* Evidence Against: *—I'm in the mall now, I was on the street then* *—There are a lot of people here, it was nearly deserted then* *—He didn't even notice me* *—He's with a girl; my assailant was alone* *—There are lots of places I could get help if I needed it here* *—He hasn't threatened me in any way*	1. Write rational response to automatic thought(s) 2. Rate belief in rational response 0–100 *It's safe here; I just got scared because he reminded me of the assailant, but that doesn't mean he's going to hurt me.* *100%*

Figure 11.3   **Sample Daily Diary PE/CR**

119 ∎

Identifying and Challenging Dysfunctional (Unhelpful) Assumptions

Once you have become good at identifying the negative beliefs that come automatically to you, cognitive therapy deals with the underlying general beliefs that we call assumptions. The major dysfunctional beliefs held by rape survivors is that the world is unsafe and they are unable to cope with stress and with their symptoms. Typical underlying assumptions for rape survivors are:

1. I must be a bad person or this wouldn't have happened to me.

2. I can't trust anybody.

3. The world is dangerous.

4. I am vulnerable.

5. I am helpless.

6. I have to be in control at all times.

7. No one is trustworthy.

You should ask yourself the following questions until you discover the underlying assumption (adapted from Clark, 1989):

1. If that thought were true, what would that mean to me?

2. What does that say about me?

3. What would happen then?

4. What would be so bad about that?

Summary for Challenging Negative Thoughts

The first step is to identify the negative thought and then challenge it. This may be hard to do on your own if you are not in therapy, but it is a skill that improves with practice. Second, look for the evidence that supports, or does not support, the negative thought. To do this, generate a list of reasons that do or do not support automatic thoughts. The third step is to review the evidence to support your thought. Have you come up with more evidence to refute the belief or to support it?

Continue to practice, complete your diary, and work on your thoughts with your therapist.

Additional Reading

Foa, E. B., & Rothbaum, B. O. (1998). *Treating the trauma of rape: Cognitive-behavioral therapy for PTSD*. New York: Guilford Press.

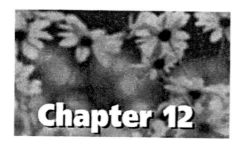

Chapter 12

Other Cognitive Techniques

About Thought-Stopping

Sometimes our thinking is troublesome in another way. Unwanted thoughts may pop into our head in a way that interferes with our functioning. Thought-stopping is a distraction technique that is used in cognitive therapy to decrease intrusive, unwanted thoughts about the assault or other distressing events. This technique is a way for you to combat a distressing thought which appears at a time that you cannot do exposure, such as in the middle of a meeting with your boss or in the middle of a party. Thought-stopping is intended for unending thinking that goes nowhere, such as obsessions, ruminations, and "crying over spilt milk." Often we do have to think about it in order to find a solution. However, when you find yourself caught in futile thinking, just looping around the same unpleasant thought or in a "why me" mood, it may be helpful to use thought-stopping to shut these thoughts off. At that point, it may be better to stop thinking about your problem. However, the use of thought-stopping for your assault-related thoughts is only temporary. In a later time during the day, you will need to come back to the thought for challenging and cognitive restructuring. Thought-stopping is a technique that you can use for relief. It is not a substitute for the careful working through discussed in the previous chapter or for imaginal exposure to the memory of the assault.

Procedure for Thought-Stopping

Following is a description of the procedure for thought-stopping. The procedure takes into consideration the fact that intrusive, unwanted thoughts can be very powerful and persistent.

Think of a disturbing thought that has been bothering you lately or keeping you up at night. Now close your eyes and focus on that thought (image). Let yourself get the thought clear in your mind. Now, shout *"Stop!"* silently in your head. Make sure you create a big racket in your head! Some people like to picture cymbals or trash can tops knocking together as they shout *"Stop!"* Remember to use some imagery, too. Many people like to picture a big, red stop sign when they shout *"Stop!"* As the stop sign goes down, it pushes the "disturbing" thoughts away and makes way for the *distracting thought*. You should have decided in your session with your therapist what your distraction will be. It can be any thought that can actively engage your mind and does not distress you. One client chose her favorite tunes from Broadway shows as her distraction. Another client used to think about interesting aspects of her job, such as her appointments for the following day. One client educated in English history would review in her head all of the kings and queens and their years in power. When all else fails, reviewing a favorite song, movie, or book is a good choice. You can always change your distraction at a later time if you need to, but change it at a time when you are *not* trying to use it. You should always know immediately what distraction to use in stopping unwanted thoughts.

Also, you may place a rubber band on your wrist and snap the rubber band lightly while silently saying *"Stop."* That often helps jolt the thought away, much as the startle of the therapist shouting *"Stop!"* If the rubber band helps, you can wear it on a regular basis, making sure it isn't too tight. If you haven't already discussed this technique with your therapist, make sure that you do now to assure that you are using this technique most effectively. It is important to understand that when using this technique it is a reminder, not a way to punish ourselves by snapping the band too hard. If this technique doesn't work for you, talk with your therapist about using another technique in its place.

Rationale for Guided Self-Dialogue

You have learned the coping skills of cognitive restructuring and thought-stopping to help you manage distressing thoughts. This section will describe guided self-dialogue, another coping skill that will help you in managing thoughts and beliefs. This skill focuses on your "self-talk," or what you are telling yourself about certain circumstances. Very often, when something is coming up that stresses us, we can make it worse by what we are telling ourselves about it. For example, if someone has a job interview coming up, at some level she may be telling herself, "They're going to laugh me out of there." Those types of negative thoughts will make her even more nervous as the time for the interview approaches. She may even cancel the interview. Those types of thoughts are not very realistic. In this example, it is unlikely the person would have applied for the job unless she thought she could do it. And it is unlikely the employer would have asked for an interview unless she looked like she could do the job. So, she may not get the job, but it is unlikely they would laugh her out of the interview. By adjusting her self-talk, she would be less anxious about the interview. This adjustment could prepare her to come across more favorably. You can now, with the assistance of your therapist, develop a list of statements that will help you control your distress before and during stressful situations.

Statements are generated in the following 4 categories:

1. Preparation for a stressor

2. Confrontation and management of a stressor

3. Coping with feelings of being overwhelmed

4. Reinforcement for coping with a stressor

For each of the categories listed above, you can generate a series of questions and/or statements to encourage you to do the following in preparing for a stressful situation:

1. Figure out what you are really scared of

2. Assess the actual probability of something terrible happening during the stressful situation

3. Manage overwhelming anxiety

4. Control self-criticism and putting yourself down

5. Do what you are scared of doing

6. Use coping self-statements

7. Pat yourself on the back for doing it

Figure 12.1 has some sample self-statements or questions in each category. You should change these and add more that would be helpful, and write them on the sheet. This technique can be used to handle everyday problems and difficulties. Sometimes it is also helpful to memorize key self-statements to use in difficult situations, and carry them with you in your purse to use in anxiety-provoking situations. Sometimes in difficult situations, our memories fail us and visual cues can help us get back on track.

There are four steps that you can take to successfully manage your reactions in stressful situations. These steps are also described in *Treating the Trauma of Rape: Cognitive-Behavioral Therapy for PTSD*. The first step is *preparing for a stressor*. In this situation, a question that you can ask yourself is "What is the likelihood that anything bad will happen?" You should try to determine, as accurately as possible, the actual probability that what you are scared of will occur. Then, try to estimate how bad it would be if it really happened. For example, it might be helpful to think in terms of a continuum of bad things.

Guided Self-Dialogue Examples

1. Preparing for a Stressor

1. What is it that I have to do?
2. What am I scared of?
3. What is the likelihood of anything bad happening?
4. How bad would it be if it really happened?
5. Don't think about how bad I feel, think about what I can do about it.
6. Don't get caught up in myself. Thinking only about my feelings won't help me cope with the situation.
7. I have the support and encouragement of people who have experience in dealing with these things.
8. I have already come a long way toward handling the problem, I can handle the rest.

List below my favorite techniques and self-statements for preparing for a stressor:

_____

_____

2. Confronting and Managing the Stressor

1. I need to take one step at a time.
2. I can handle this.
3. Don't think about how afraid or anxious I am, think about what I am doing. The feeling that I am having now is a signal for me to use my coping exercises.
4. There is no need to doubt myself. I have the skills I need to get through this.
5. Focus on my plan. Relax and take a calming breath. I am ready to go.

List below your favorite techniques and self-statements for confronting and handling a stressor:

_____

_____

3. Coping with Feelings of Being Overwhelmed

1. When I feel afraid, I will take a breath and exhale slowly, saying to myself "calm."
2. Focus on what is happening now; what is it that I have to do?
3. I can expect my fear to rise but I can keep it manageable.
4. This fear may slow me down but it will not stop me.
5. Think to myself "this will pass and it will be over soon."
6. I may feel scared and anxious but I can do it.

List below your favorite techniques and self-statements for coping with feelings of being overwhelmed:

_____

_____

4. Reinforcement for Managing a Stressor

1. It was much easier than I thought.
2. I did it—I got through it and each time will be easier.
3. When I manage my thoughts in my head, I can manage the feelings in my body.
4. I am making progress.
5. I did a good job.
6. One step at a time.

Generate a list of your favorite positive statements for reinforcing managing with a stressor:

_____

_____

Figure 12.1.

"0" might be something like breaking a fingernail or mildly stubbing a toe: it's not great, but in the scheme of things it is insignificant. "100" might be something like serious harm or death to you or a loved one. Weigh both the probability of the bad thing, and how bad it would be if the bad thing really happened.

It is also helpful to defocus on your anxiety at this point. There are statements to try to help you do this. When we get into "woe is me" thinking, focusing on how bad we feel, it tends to make us feel worse and doesn't help in any way. For example, if you are getting ready for something you're very excited about and you stub your toe, you almost don't notice it. Whereas, if you've had a lousy day and are tired and depressed and stub your toe, you could almost sit down and cry about it. The actual pain is no worse in one situation or the other. What differs is your degree of focus on it.

The second step is *confronting and managing a stressor*. These self-statements are helpful in managing the anxiety that you anticipate before the stressful situation happens. For example, you are sitting at home worrying about going to work the next morning. Quite often, your anticipatory anxiety is far worse than the anxiety that you experience once you have entered a situation. These statements will help you manage your anxious thoughts. Very often, people react to anxiety with more anxiety. When they notice themselves getting tense, they think, "Oh, no! Here it comes again. I can't handle this. This is terrible." All this does is make them more anxious. These coping statements and this program will try to let you use your anxiety as a cue to use coping strategies to manage it. For example, when you notice your heart racing, use it as a cue to use your breathing technique to slow it down.

The third step is *coping with feelings of being overwhelmed*. You are learning techniques to reduce this anxiety while you are in the stressful situation. An example of this would be ways to help when you actually go into your work place and start to feel anxious and uncomfortable. We like for people to remind themselves that if they have chosen to be in this situation, that usually means they can handle it. We very rarely choose to put ourselves in situations we can't handle. (Note: people don't choose to be assaulted, even if they chose to be in that location.) The situation may be challenging, but if we have decided to do it, we usually can.

The fourth step is *reinforcing self-statements*. It's important to pat yourself on the back when you have done something that was stressful for you. It is appropriate to praise a child who has done something that was difficult for her no matter how she actually did. You deserve praise for doing things that are difficult for you as well. What do you usually say to yourself when you've done well?

Before starting to learn this stress-management procedure, review each step to identify the self-statements that will be most helpful to you. As you go through the statements, feel free to add any of your favorite self-statements to each list. Also, if you dislike any of these statements, or feel they don't apply to you, scratch them out. First, apply this to a non-assault-related example. Think of a stressful event coming up that is not related to the assault.

Non-Assault-Related Stressful Events Examples

- Calling a friend who is mad with you

- Preparing dinner for an important person or group

- Asking for a raise at work

After developing self-statements and coping strategies to cope with a non-assault situation, go on to an assault-related situation.

Assault-Related Stressful Events Examples

- Being alone at home

- Going to the mall alone

- Talking with people about the assault

- Going out on a date

- Going to your gynecologist for annual exam

- Testifying against the assailant at trial

As always, keep practicing these techniques!

Additional Reading

Foa, E. B., & Rothbaum, B. O. (1998). *Treating the trauma of rape: Cognitive-behavioral therapy for PTSD*. New York: Guilford Press.

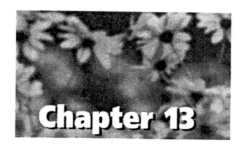

Chapter 13

Role-play, Assertive Behavior, and Covert Modeling

About Role-play

A technique called role-play will help you learn new behaviors and words to use in situations that make you anxious. Have you ever had the experience of role-playing before? Role-playing is like a dress rehearsal. This technique is based on the principle that practicing what you want to say before you enter a stressful situation helps to decrease your anxiety and gives you a higher chance of obtaining your goal. If you are in therapy, your therapist can role-play with you in session. Here is how it works.

Some role-plays will deal with how to be more assertive. Assertiveness is saying what you need to say in an effective way. One important point is that being assertive is not the same as being aggressive. Think about assertiveness as the happy medium between being passive and being aggressive. If a person is passive all the time and lets people walk all over her, she may become angry and explode over minor incidents. This isn't a helpful way to act with family, friends, or coworkers. On the other hand, if a person is aggressive with someone, she may initially get what she wants, but in the long run people may start avoiding her. Let's talk about the difference between aggressive, nonassertive, and assertive behaviors.

Aggressive behavior is denying someone else their rights and feelings by blaming them, name-calling, or using other behaviors that are designed to get your way no matter what, even though it may hurt them or make them feel defensive.

Nonassertive or *passive behavior* is denying your own rights by not standing up for yourself or not expressing your feelings. It can also include indirect communication (e.g. body language) that is easy to misinterpret.

Assertive behavior does not violate your rights or someone else's rights. Assertive behavior is expressing your feelings and preferences in a direct, honest, and appropriate manner. Assertive behavior conveys respect for other people's feelings and facilitates two-way communication. It often involves making compromises. Being assertive involves using specific words, behaviors, and body postures. Table 13.1 presents a list of assertive behaviors that you may want to write down on index cards to make it more accessible to review frequently.

Table 13.1.   Assertive Communication

The following is a list of helpful hints when you are trying to communicate an important message to someone:

1. Maintain eye contact and when you take breaks, move your eyes to the side

    a. moving eyes up makes you look bored

    b. moving eyes down makes you look shy or insecure

2. Keep your facial expression appropriate to the message that you are sending

3. Maintain an erect, not rigid or slumped, body posture

    a. sit up straight

    b. keep hands and arms by side

    c. do not cross arms or wring hands

    d. position of body should face listener

4. Voice tone should be even, inflection and volume should be normal

    a. don't yell, scream, or speak too loudly

    b. don't speak too softly

    c. don't cry

5. Content of statements should be brief and to the point

    a. it is helpful to tell listener what you expect them to do (e.g., "I would like to talk with you about something very important and then I would like to hear your feedback" or "I am hoping that you will be able to help me with something")

6. Find the right moment to talk

    a. don't catch someone who is running off somewhere

    b. don't interrupt a conversation

    c. don't demand to speak to someone immediately

Assertive behaviors include the following:

a. Maintain eye contact with the person with whom you are talking.

b. Your facial expression should be appropriate to the message you are sending (e.g., do not smile when you are telling someone you are upset by something that they did).

c. Your body posture should be erect (not rigid or slumped).

d. Do not fidget with your hands, wring hands, or sit with legs and arms crossed.

e. Your voice tone, inflection, and volume should be normal (don't yell, whine, cry or whisper).

f. The content of your statements should be brief and direct; do not accuse, blame, or be defensive.

g. Timing is essential. Plan ahead to have a conversation and don't catch someone if he or she is running off to a meeting or engaged in an activity that requires concentration.

h. When you are telling someone something that is hard for you to say or may be hard for them to hear, it is helpful to use the following 4 "parts":

    1) Start with something positive (e.g., "Honey, you know that I love you.")

    2) Say exactly what it was that they did (e.g., "When you come up behind me and surprise me by hugging me. . .")

    3) Say exactly the effect on you (e.g., "It startles me and leaves me very rattled.")

    4) Say exactly what you would like from them in the future (e.g., "So, I would appreciate it if you could warn me before you hug me from behind so I don't get startled.")

During the role-play training, you and your therapist will actually act out scenes of a situation that you anticipate will be disturbing. Role-playing is the acting out of behaviors, rehearsing of lines and actions, and pretending to be in a specific set of circumstances. Role-playing is a way to learn new behaviors and words for expressing your needs and intentions more clearly before the event occurs. Like a dress rehearsal, the repeated practice of a behavior reduces anxiety and makes it more likely that a new behavior will be used. Role-plays can be repeated until you perform the behaviors well or level off. This practice rarely requires more than 5 times. When you are practicing at home, you can ask a friend or relative to role-play with you. The following presents some non-assault and assault-related situations to role play:

Examples of Non-Assault-Related Situations For Role-play

- Talking to your boss
- Requesting time off from your boss
- Asking for an escort to walk you to your car in the parking garage
- Asking significant others to assist you with in vivo exposure exercises
- Calling a friend to ask if you can borrow something
- Saying "no" to an authority figure

Examples of Assault-Related Situations For Role-play

- Telling a family member about the assault
- Walking in a calm and confident manner
- Using assertive body language when making a point
- Saying "no" to a sexual interaction
- Saying "no" to a request to go on a date at night with an unfamiliar man
- Telling someone who approaches you and talks that you don't want to talk to them

Case Example of Assertive Feedback

Mary was a 34-year-old married woman who was raped at knifepoint in her car after having to drive the assailant from the mall to an abandoned lot. Her husband tried to be supportive and clearly loved Mary, but had a difficult time with the idea of the assault, particularly that another man had "violated" his wife. Mary felt that he didn't want to hear anything about the assault, and, in fact, he would change the subject or encourage her "to forget about it" if she did bring it up. Besides feeling the need to talk about it herself, her husband's reaction made Mary uncomfortable and led her to feel dirty and guilty. Mary brought this issue up when discussing role-play and decided she would like to talk to her husband about it but wasn't sure how. First, the therapist played Mary and had Mary play her husband. The dialogue is represented with **T** signifying the *Therapist* and **M** signifying *Mary*:

T: (as Mary) Lou, do you have a few minutes now?

M: (as her husband) Sure, honey. What's up?

T: (as Mary) Lou, you know I love you and I think you're a great husband. You've tried to take care of me after this whole rape thing, and I appreciate it.

M: (as her husband) Awww, do we have to talk about that again?

T: (as Mary) Just bear with me a minute: this is hard for me.

M: (as her husband) Okay, sorry.

T: (as Mary) I know the rape was hard on you, too. And I know you don't like to talk about it. But when you change the subject when I bring it up, or when you get so uncomfortable when it comes up, it makes me feel even worse, like you can't even look at me and think what happened to me. It makes me feel dirty and alone and like you wish you weren't married to me anymore.

[Mary had said these things to the therapist.]

M: (as her husband) It's just that I can't stand to think what that scum did to you.

T: (as Mary) I know, but just not thinking about it doesn't make it go away. I need to talk to you about it, and I need for you to feel more comfortable hearing and talking about it.

M: (as her husband) I don't know how to do that.

T: (as Mary) We can start by just talking more about it, even when it gets uncomfortable. And I'd like it if you let me talk about it when I bring it up. And I'd love it if you could talk about it more and tell me what you're feeling and thinking. What do you think of this?

M: (as her husband) I'm willing to try if you think it will help you.

Mary and the therapist then discussed aspects in the therapist's behavior that Mary liked: she liked the words the therapist used; she liked how the therapist didn't drop it when the husband tried to change the subject; Mary also liked the therapist's nonverbal signals, she thought her facial expression and posture gave the message that she wasn't going to back down and this was important. The therapist asked Mary for feedback on things to improve: Mary felt her husband would respond positively to her request to allow her to talk but didn't know how he would respond to her request for him to share his feelings, but she decided it was worth a try to ask him anyway. Then, they reversed roles with Mary playing herself and the therapist playing Mary's husband. Mary had some difficulty at first, especially spitting out what she wanted to say and using appropriate nonverbal signals. After two repetitions, Mary had it down, feeling comfortable and confident and determined to go home and have that conversation that evening, which she did.

About Covert Modeling

Another coping skill that is somewhat similar to role-playing is called "covert modeling" which just means role-playing in your imagination. This activity is covert, or imagined, rather than overt, out in the open, like actual role-plays. This technique involves modeling, or picturing someone else going through the situation first. It will help you manage situations in which you feel anxious and uncomfortable. The goal is to bring up problems that you can visualize in your imagination, and first picture someone else going through it successfully. Then, pull them out and substitute yourself going through it just the way they did, like following in their footsteps.

We practice coping so when the situation or a similar situation comes up, you will have successfully practiced dealing with it. Again, the technique is a bit different than role-playing because you will first imagine someone else coping with the stressor, then imagine yourself doing the same, not rehearsing it by interacting with anyone. This technique is necessary when a person can't even imagine themselves doing something, or doing it again after the assault. For example, one woman couldn't even imagine getting through a job interview. When asked if she had a friend she *could* imagine getting through a job interview, she recalled a friend that she was sure could do it. By imagining her friend doing it first, she could delineate all steps involved and what would be required for a successful outcome. Then, it was easier to pluck her friend out of the picture and imagine herself doing what was necessary to do it. This is similar to positive visualization, like when the golfer pictures the ball going into the hole before she putts it. As usual, practice with a non-assault-related example to rehearse, then practice it with an assault-related example. You should close your eyes to aid imagery, but you can practice the imagery with your eyes open if you feel uncomfortable about closing them.

Examples of Assault-Related Situations For Covert Modeling

- Being on date and the male makes sexual advances

- Being on date and being anxious in presence of man

- Walking home from a train station

- Leaving work to go to the car

- Going to public places (e.g., grocery store, mall, restaurant, movie theater)

- Sexual interaction with partner

- Talking with co-workers who are making jokes about a woman who was raped

Practice with your therapist first by using a non-assault example and then applying the technique to an assault-related example.

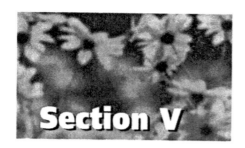

Section V

Cognitive-Behavioral Program

Putting It All Together

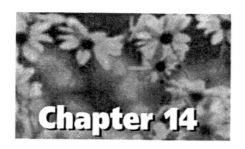

Chapter 14

Putting the Techniques Together: Common Problems and Complications

Checking Progress

At the end of Session 8, it is time to check your progress in treatment and to evaluate whether or not you need more sessions. At this time, your therapist may have asked you to complete some of the questionnaires and interviews again. If so, please use this information in evaluating your progress in the program.

You may remember rating your PTSD symptoms previously in Chapter 5. We would like for you to re-assess your PTSD symptoms at this point. Below is a description of the PTSD symptoms. Please rate each symptom that you are *currently* experiencing on a 0—3 scale. "0" indicates that you do not have this symptom or that it is so mild that it is not at all a problem for you; "1" indicates it is a mild problem for you; "2" indicates it is a moderate problem for you; and "3" indicates it is a severe problem for you:

> **0 = not a problem**
>
> **1 = mild problem**
>
> **2 = moderate problem**
>
> **3 = severe problem**

I. Reexperiencing the traumatic event:

___ 1. Thoughts, images, or ideas about the trauma that keep coming back and are unwanted and cause distress

___ 2. Nightmares or bad dreams about the trauma or that seem related to it

_____ 3. Flashbacks of the traumatic event, as if it were happening again

_____ 4. Extreme emotional distress when I am reminded of the traumatic event

_____ 5. Extreme bodily reactions when I am reminded of the traumatic event (for example, heart races, get sweaty, tense up)

II. Continual avoidance of reminders of the traumatic event and/or emotional numbing:

_____ 1. Avoid thinking about, talking about, or feelings associated with the trauma

_____ 2. Avoid situations, activities, places, or people that remind me of the traumatic event

_____ 3. Can't remember _important_ parts of what happened

_____ 4. Large decrease in interest or time spent in activities that were important to me

_____ 5. Feeling cut off from or like I can't connect with other people

_____ 6. Emotional numbing; don't experience the whole range of emotions that I used to

_____ 7. Feel my life will be cut short; don't expect to live as long as I had thought

III. Indications of increased arousal:

_____ 1. Continual problems falling or staying asleep

_____ 2. Extreme irritability or outbursts of anger

_____ 3. Persistent difficulty concentrating

_____ 4. Extreme "scanning" of environment, checking the situation all around me, hypervigilant

_____ 5. Extremely jumpy, startle very easily

Compare your current ratings to your previous ratings in Chapter 5. We generally suggest that clients who have not improved very much on their PTSD symptoms receive 3 additional treatment sessions. If there are clear and ongoing reasons why you did not improve more (e.g., if you are in the middle of the trial or are receiving threatening phone calls), and if you think additional sessions would not be useful at this time, you may want to end your treatment now. You can also discuss with the therapist the possibility of additional sessions in the future when you may be able to profit more from them. Another therapeutic option is to stop focusing on reducing your PTSD symptoms at this time and focus instead on receiving support from your therapist if this is a difficult period. You can resume cognitive-behavioral work at a later point. You and your therapist should carefully consider your progress and therapeutic options together.

Some questions to help determine your progress:

1. How are you feeling now compared to when you began the program?

2. What have you learned?

3. What were the most helpful techniques?

4. Was there anything that you didn't find very helpful?

5. Are there any skills that you think you need to continue to practice?

As a reminder, below is a list of the techniques you may have used and what they are designed to help with:

1. Imaginal and in vivo exposure—help you confront the memory of the assault and reminders of it with less discomfort

2. Breathing, deep muscle, and differential relaxation—help you learn to relax your body

3. Thought-stopping—helps you learn to distract yourself from thoughts that cause you distress and are not useful to you

4. Cognitive restructuring—helps you think more logically, rationally

5. Preparing for a stressor—helps you use coping self-talk in stressful situations

6. Covert modeling and role-play—help you be able to say and do what you would like

In your opinion, do you feel you need more treatment? If yes, for what types of issues? What are some potential difficulties or stressful situations that may arise in the future? Can you plan ways to manage these situations effectively using some of these techniques? You may want to discuss these ideas with your therapist and note the discussion in your diary, so you can refer to it later.

If you have used this program by this time you have probably spent quite a lot of time doing in vivo exposure exercises to help you approach people and situations that became scary for you after the assault. You have been processing your traumatic memories by repeatedly reliving the assault and recounting it aloud in sessions and during homework. You have learned a variety of coping skills to help decrease your anxiety in stressful situations or challenging thoughts that brought about intense negative emotions. You have learned cognitive restructuring that included learning to identify, challenge, and modify negative thoughts and assumptions that you were having because of the assault and that caused intense emotional reactions. Other techniques were thought-stopping, relaxation, and role-playing and covert modeling.

Have you noticed any changes in your thoughts or feelings as a result of the treatment and learning the coping skills? Specifically what are those?

_____
_____
_____
_____
_____

What have you noticed about your level of anxiety or discomfort in certain situations?

_____
_____
_____
_____
_____

What skills have you found most helpful to manage that anxiety and discomfort?

_____
_____
_____
_____
_____

Are there any problems that you are still concerned about? If so, discuss these with your therapist for his or her professional recommendation.

_____
_____
_____
_____
_____

Common Problems and Complications

Following is a discussion of issues that can complicate your therapy. It is important to understand these issues if they are preventing you from making progress in therapy.

Avoidance/Resistance

PTSD assault survivors may be especially resistant to engaging emotionally in treatment. There are several reasons for this. First, their trauma is an interpersonal injury caused by an intentionally malicious act that another person directed at them. Therefore, they may have less trust in fellow humans. Secondly, they have a tendency to use avoidant coping mechanisms during exposure treatment. The survivor is asked to perform two extremely difficult tasks: to intentionally expose herself to the very memory she has been actively avoiding, and to trust the therapist to assist her throughout this difficult and challenging experience. The difficulty of trusting combined with the tendency on the part of many PTSD assault survivors to avoid emotional engagement with the traumatic memory results in reluctance to emotionally engage during reliving sessions. Even when a survivor is recounting the details of her assault, she may be emotionally distancing herself, appearing to tell someone else's story rather than her own. This reluctance to engage emotionally can hinder treatment because studies have shown a relationship between emotional responses during imaginal reliving of the trauma and benefit from treatment. The third issue important to exposure therapy with rape survivors stems from the intimate nature of the rape trauma. This may result in much difficulty in telling someone else the details of the assault. It is less embarrassing to discuss an attack by a dog than to discuss details of being raped. You must trust that your therapist can handle the details. She or he would not be doing this type of therapy if they could not handle it.

Actual Risk

Another issue specific to assault survivors is the extreme care in selecting situations for in vivo self-exposure. You and your therapist must carefully assess the realistic probability for harm during exposure in vivo. Indeed, in some environments assaults may be quite frequent. Some of our clients were continually threatened or harassed by their assailants. In these cases, it may be necessary for your therapist to help you to involve the police and obtain a restraining order to keep the assailant away from you. The first order of business is to insure your safety. A shelter or temporary residence may also be considered, if necessary. Shelters are safe havens available in many communities for women and children who are at risk.

Decision making guidelines for the use of exposure therapy for PTSD have been established and take into account client's variables such as tolerance for extreme arousal, imagery ability, and compliance (see the 1996 Jaycox and Foa article for more information). Clearly, women who are experiencing extreme distress when remembering their assault or show extreme avoidance of situations, objects, or thoughts which remind them of it, would profit from exposure therapy. However, for some assault survivors the memories are excruciatingly painful, resulting in resistance to comply with exposure instructions. In these extreme cases, you may need to take a more gradual approach or begin your therapy with anxiety management techniques before exposure.

Compliance

It is very important for you to keep regular appointments, even if you are inclined to avoid them. You need to face this to get through it. Push yourself now; it will be worth it!

Sticking with the program, particularly in homework practice, can be a problem. The treatment program we have presented in this book requires considerable time outside of the therapy session. You must practice anxiety management skills several times daily and expose yourself imaginally and in vivo daily as well. If you are not practicing as prescribed, please discuss this with your therapist. Try to problem solve. If you don't seem to have the time to practice between work and taking care of home and the family, go through your daily schedule with your therapist. Hopefully, together you can see where you can grab some time for yourself. This may require help from a partner or a support person to take up your slack and, for example, watch the kids after supper while you practice. The stress management techniques are all skills that must be practiced to be mastered and used effectively, and exposure requires repeated listening to the tape or practicing of in vivo exercises to allow the necessary changes to take place. In other words, you must do your homework!

If you are continuously unable to put the necessary time into this treatment, you may need to terminate treatment at this point. *Timing* is very important. When it is the right time to deal with a problem, you will invest in your treatment and benefit from it. When it is not the right time, even potentially effective techniques will not be helpful and you will become frustrated. If you cannot give priority to the treatment exercises then it may not be the right time for you to be in this treatment right now. We would rather have you stop early, knowing you did not have a complete program, than have you plod along, be frustrated with the lack of progress, and get the idea that nothing can help you. The bottom line is that we do not think you are going to achieve all that you could if you do not practice sufficiently between sessions. Therefore, it may be best to stop treatment at this point and come back to it later when you are able to devote more time and energy to it. When the right time comes for you, you can call this same therapist if you feel comfortable. If, when you're ready, you think you might like to try again but with a different therapist, that is what you should do. Most therapists are aware that they may not be the best match for everyone and may help you find someone else to work with. The most important thing is that the timing and the therapist be right for you.

Lack of Support

Many clients will require outside support to enter into and complete this program. This includes emotional support and encouragement to face the traumatic memories during treatment. It also includes logistical support (e.g., child care) to make it possible to attend sessions and complete homework. If you have a partner who is not supportive, it can greatly interfere with therapy. Often, husbands or boyfriends may not understand PTSD and its treatment and/or might not think it is important. You can help educate them by letting them read the "Common Reactions to Assault" part of this workbook or having a session with the therapist. Some clients have wanted their partners to listen to the tape of the imaginal exposure so that they could know what they went through. Explaining to your partner your reactions and your need for treatment may be role-played with your therapist so you can communicate this more easily. Also, you may want to consider support groups for partners of rape survivors in your area.

It is also important to be watchful of your partner's discomfort with the treatment and with the changes that you may go through in treatment. We have seen clients whose relationships were built on the survivor's dependency on her partner. If in treatment the client starts getting more independent, adventuresome, and confident, she may want to change the dependency aspect of the relationship. This may be very threatening to the partner, who is used to this arrangement, and may need to be addressed as a part of treatment. Couples can be directed to grow together rather than apart. If this is the case with you and your partner, you may profit from couples therapy, or you may want to bring him to your session and discuss these issues together with your therapist.

Other Disorders

Many assault survivors suffer from other psychological problems in addition to PTSD, as previously discussed. Substance abuse is particularly high in PTSD sufferers. Many PTSD sufferers use drugs and alcohol to self-medicate themselves to reduce the emotional pain associated with the trauma. It is quite clear that substance abuse needs to be addressed before or simultaneously with treatment for the PTSD, because substance abuse will interfere with the necessary emotional processing. It is best to be clean and sober for about 90 days before treating assault-related issues. As mentioned earlier, if this is a problem for you, you should seek counseling for substance abuse.

Many PTSD assault survivors are mildly to moderately depressed. As we discussed in Chapter 3, if you are suffering from a severe major depression, the depression should be treated before the PTSD. In this case, antidepressant medications, psychosocial treatments, or inpatient hospitalization may be indicated. On the other hand, mild or moderate depression should not pose a problem to treatment and would be expected to respond favorably to the treatment outlined in this book.

Your problems must be prioritized with the most severe, threatening, and disruptive ones being addressed first. Suicidal tendencies obviously take priority. We have found this treatment program to be quite effective and manageable with clients who suffered from problems other than PTSD, as long as the other problems are known and dealt with. You and your therapist should discuss these issues if they exist for you.

Additional Reading

Jaycox, L. H., & Foa, E. B. (1996). Obstacles in implementing exposure therapy for PTSD: Case discussions and practical solutions. *Clinical Psychology and Psychotherapy, 3*(3), 176-184.

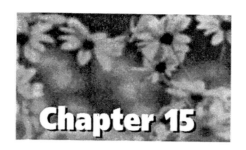

Chapter 15

Where Do I Go From Here?

Hopefully, by this point, you have made it through the therapy program. We hope you have found it helpful. Where do you go from here?

Do you feel you made good progress in this program? Does your therapist agree? If so, it sounds like you may be ready to terminate treatment. We discussed in Chapter 14 how to determine if you would benefit from more sessions. You can use that evaluation to help determine the best road for you now. Even if you feel you responded well to this program, you can identify areas that you need to continue to work on. Now, you can decide which of the techniques were most helpful to you and continue to use them when you work on these areas. It is highly likely you can do it on your own. You may use this client workbook for your continued self-work.

If you decide that you still have a lot of problems that you need to work on, think about why you did not achieve more with this program. Was this the right time in your life to be working on your assault-related problems? If not, we recommend you try again with these same techniques when it feels more like the right time. Was this the right type of program for you? If you don't think so, we urge you to discuss this with your therapist. She or he can help determine what type of treatment would best meet your needs now. Have you tried as hard as you could to get the most out of this program? Did obstacles interfere? Did you practice regularly? Were you as motivated as you could have been? If not, it may be best to try again when you feel the time is right and your motivation is high. You may return to sections of this workbook that were difficult for you when the time is right.

Whatever gains you may have achieved in this program, it is important to maintain those gains. Think about your habits before treatment that maintained your problems, and think about how you are doing things differently now. You must keep doing things the new way. You must not let yourself slip back into avoiding, which is one of the behaviors that maintained your initial symptoms. Don't avoid doing things or going places if they are safe just because they remind you of the assault. Don't avoid talking or thinking about the assault. Continue practicing the stress management techniques that were helpful. Continue using the imaginal exposure while listening to the tape. It is also important to fill your life with rewarding activities and people. Get back to living a full life. Set goals for yourself at work and at home and work towards those. You might want to list and check on positive goals for yourself on a regular basis.

Try to plan ahead for high-risk times in the future. By "high-risk," we mean times that make you vulnerable for relapse or experience problems again. For example, if your assailant is caught and prosecuted, the trial is usually a very stressful time for assault survivors. The anniversary of the assault is another such time. Another example of a high-risk time might be if your partner needed to start traveling more for work, leaving you at home alone more. If you can anticipate situations that might cause you difficulty, you can prepare yourself and handle them better. Try not to let these situations take you by surprise, but, if they do, try to use these new skills to bounce back quickly.

Congratulations on completing this program and hopefully gaining some peace of mind. We wish you luck, endurance, safety, health, love, and laughter in your life.

Breinigsville, PA USA
12 October 2010

247116BV00002B/1/P